INTRODUCTION

D ementia is a progressive and multifaceted neurological condition characterized by a decline in cognitive abilities, including memory, reasoning, and the ability to perform daily activities. As the global population ages, the prevalence of dementia continues to rise, presenting significant challenges for individuals, families, and healthcare systems. While there is currently no cure for dementia, emerging research suggests that lifestyle factors, including diet, may play a crucial role in supporting cognitive health and potentially mitigating the risk of cognitive decline.

The brain, an organ highly susceptible to the effects of aging and various diseases, relies on a complex interplay of nutrients for optimal function. Consequently, attention to dietary habits has become a focal point in exploring avenues for promoting brain health and potentially delaying the onset of cognitive disorders such as dementia. This recognition has given rise to a growing body of research investigating the impact of specific nutrients, dietary patterns, and lifestyle choices on cognitive function and the progression of dementia.

The role of diet in dementia is multifaceted,

encompassing various aspects of nutrition that influence brain health. Certain dietary patterns, such as the Mediterranean diet, have gained prominence for their potential neuroprotective effects. Rich in fruits, vegetables, whole grains, and healthy fats, this diet is associated with a reduced risk of cognitive decline. Furthermore, specific nutrients, such as omega-3 fatty acids found in fatty fish and antioxidants present in colorful fruits and vegetables, have garnered attention for their potential to combat oxidative stress and inflammation, processes implicated in the pathogenesis of dementia.

CHAPTER ONE

Definition of Dementia

Dementia is a broad and complex term used to describe a group of progressive neurological disorders characterized by a decline in cognitive function that goes beyond what is considered a normal part of aging. It is not a specific disease but rather a syndrome with various causes, each affecting the brain differently. The hallmark feature of dementia is a deterioration in cognitive abilities, impacting memory, reasoning, language, and the ability to carry out everyday activities.

TYPES OF DEMENTIA

Dementia encompasses a spectrum of neurological disorders, each with its unique characteristics, causes, and progression patterns. Here is a comprehensive overview of five common types of dementia:

1. Alzheimer's Disease:

• Description: Alzheimer's disease is the most prevalent form of dementia, accounting for a significant majority of cases. It is a progressive neurodegenerative disorder characterized by the accumulation of abnormal protein deposits, including beta-amyloid plaques and tau tangles, in the brain.

• Symptoms: Memory loss, cognitive decline, impaired reasoning and judgment, changes in behavior and personality.

• Progression: Alzheimer's disease typically progresses slowly over several years, with early stages marked by mild memory lapses and later stages leading to severe impairment in daily functioning.

1. Vascular Dementia:

• Description: Vascular dementia results from impaired blood flow to the brain, often due to stroke or other vascular issues. The damage can be widespread or occur in specific regions of the brain.

• Symptoms: Cognitive decline, difficulties with organization and planning, problems with attention and concentration.

• Progression: The progression of vascular dementia can vary, with symptoms often appearing suddenly after a stroke or gradually worsening over time. It may coexist with other forms of dementia, such as Alzheimer's disease.

1. Lewy Body Dementia:

• Description: Lewy's body dementia is characterized by the presence of abnormal protein deposits called Lewy's bodies in the brain. It shares features with both Alzheimer's disease and Parkinson's disease.

• Symptoms: Fluctuating cognitive abilities, visual hallucinations, motor symptoms similar to Parkinson's disease, sleep disturbances.

• Progression: Lewy body dementia often progresses gradually, with a combination of cognitive, motor, and psychiatric symptoms that can be challenging to manage.

1. Frontotemporal Dementia:

• Description: Frontotemporal dementia involves degeneration of the frontal and temporal lobes of the brain, affecting behavior, personality, and language.

• Symptoms: Changes in personality, social behavior, language difficulties, and executive function impairment.

• Progression: Frontotemporal dementia tends to have a more rapid onset than Alzheimer's disease, with distinct behavioral and language variants. It often occurs in individuals under the age of 65.

1. Mixed Dementia:

• Description: Mixed dementia refers to the coexistence of multiple types of dementia, most commonly Alzheimer's disease and vascular dementia. This combination can complicate the clinical presentation and progression.

• Symptoms: A mix of symptoms associated with the different types of dementia present.

• Progression: The progression of mixed dementia depends on the combination of underlying causes, with symptoms reflecting a blend of cognitive, motor, and behavioral impairments.

CAUSES AND RISK FACTORS

Dementia is a complex and multifactorial syndrome with various causes and risk factors contributing to its onset and progression. Understanding these factors is crucial for both prevention strategies and providing targeted interventions for those affected. Here are the causes and risk factors associated with dementia:

1. Age:
    a. Cause: Age is the most significant risk factor for dementia. The prevalence of dementia increases with advancing age, and the risk rises substantially in individuals over the age of 65.
    b. Explanation: The aging process itself can lead to changes in the brain, including the accumulation of abnormal proteins, reduced neurotransmitter function, and diminished brain volume.
2. Genetics:
    a. Cause: Genetic factors play a role in certain types of dementia, with a family history of the condition increasing the risk.

    b. Explanation: Mutations in specific genes, such as those associated with Alzheimer's disease or frontotemporal dementia, can contribute to an increased likelihood of developing dementia. However, familial cases represent a minority, and most dementia cases occur sporadically.

3. Cardiovascular Health:

    a. Cause: Poor cardiovascular health and conditions that affect blood flow to the brain can contribute to the development of vascular dementia.

    b. Explanation: Hypertension, atherosclerosis, heart disease, and conditions leading to strokes can impair blood circulation to the brain, resulting in damage to brain tissue and an increased risk of dementia.

4. Lifestyle Factors:

    a. Cause: Certain lifestyle factors have been linked to an increased or decreased risk of dementia.

    b. Explanation:

    c. Physical Inactivity: Lack of regular physical exercise is associated with a higher risk of dementia. Physical activity promotes cardiovascular health and has neuroprotective effects on the brain.

    d. Dietary Habits: Poor dietary choices, such as a high intake of saturated fats sugars, and low intake of fruits and vegetables, may contribute to an increased risk of dementia. Conversely, a diet rich in antioxidants and omega-3 fatty acids may have protective effects.

e. Smoking: Smoking is a recognized risk factor for dementia, likely due to its impact on cardiovascular health and the brain's susceptibility to oxidative stress.

f. Alcohol Consumption: Excessive alcohol consumption has been linked to an increased risk of dementia. Moderate alcohol intake, however, may have a protective effect.

g. Cognitive Stimulation: Engaging in mentally stimulating activities, such as reading, learning, and social interactions, is associated with a reduced risk of cognitive decline.

SYMPTOMS OF DEMENTIA

Dementia is characterized by a range of symptoms that reflect a decline in cognitive function, affecting various aspects of an individual's daily life. The symptoms can vary depending on the type of dementia and the specific areas of the brain involved. Here are the common symptoms associated with dementia:

1. Memory Loss:
    a. Description: One of the hallmark symptoms of dementia is progressive memory loss. Individuals may need help recalling recent events, forgetting names, and need help remembering familiar faces.
2. Cognitive Decline:
    a. Description: Dementia often leads to a decline in overall cognitive abilities. Individuals may experience difficulties in reasoning, problem-solving, and making decisions. They may also need help with concentrating and following conversations.
3. Impaired Communication:
    a. Description: Dementia can affect

language skills, leading to difficulties in expressing thoughts, finding the right words, or understanding spoken or written language. Communication breakdowns may result in frustration and social withdrawal.

4. Disorientation:
   a. Description: Individuals with dementia may become disoriented in time and space. They may need to keep track of dates, seasons, and the passage of time. Getting lost in familiar places is also a common occurrence.

5. Behavioral Changes:
   a. Description: Dementia often brings about changes in behavior and personality. Individuals may exhibit mood swings, increased irritability, anxiety, depression, or apathy. Social withdrawal and a loss of interest in once-enjoyed activities can occur.

6. Difficulty Performing Daily Tasks:
   a. Description: As dementia progresses, individuals may struggle to perform routine tasks, such as dressing, grooming, or preparing meals. The ability to handle finances and manage medications may also be compromised.

7. Impaired Motor Skills:
   a. Description: Some types of dementia, such as Lewy body dementia, may affect motor skills, leading to stiffness, tremors, or difficulties with

coordination and balance.

8. Poor Judgment:
   a. Description: Dementia can impair an individual's judgment and decision-making abilities. This may manifest as poor financial choices, risky behaviors, or an inability to assess the consequences of actions.

9. Hallucinations and Delusions:
   a. Description: In certain types of dementia, particularly Lewy body dementia, individuals may experience visual hallucinations and delusions, which can be distressing for both the affected individual and their caregivers.

10. Sleep Disturbances:
    a. Description: Changes in sleep patterns are common in dementia. Individuals may experience insomnia, daytime drowsiness, or disturbances in the sleep-wake cycle.

DIAGNOSIS OF DEMENTIA

Diagnosing dementia involves a comprehensive evaluation that considers a person's medical history, cognitive function, and, in some cases, neuroimaging studies. The process is often intricate, and an accurate diagnosis is crucial for guiding appropriate care and support. Here is an overview of the steps and considerations involved in the diagnosis of dementia:

1. Clinical Assessment:
    a. Medical History: A thorough medical history is essential to identify any underlying medical conditions, medications, or family history of dementia. Certain medical conditions, such as vitamin deficiencies or thyroid dysfunction, can contribute to cognitive impairment.
2. Cognitive Assessment:
    a. Mini-Mental State Examination (MMSE): This widely used tool assesses cognitive function, including memory, attention, and language. It helps quantify the severity of cognitive impairment and track changes over time.

    b. Montreal Cognitive Assessment (MoCA): Similar to the MMSE, the MoCA evaluates various cognitive domains, including memory, language, and executive function, providing a more detailed assessment.

3. Neurological Examination:

    a. Evaluation of Motor Skills: A neurological examination assesses motor skills, coordination, and reflexes. This can help identify signs of specific types of dementia, such as Parkinsonism in Lewy body dementia.

4. Blood Tests:

    a. Routine Blood Tests: Blood tests are conducted to rule out reversible causes of cognitive impairment, such as vitamin deficiencies, thyroid dysfunction, or metabolic disorders.

5. Neuroimaging Studies:

    a. MRI (Magnetic Resonance Imaging): An MRI scan provides detailed images of the brain and can help identify structural changes, such as atrophy or the presence of lesions.

    b. CT (Computed Tomography) Scan: CT scans may be used to assess brain structure and rule out conditions like tumors or bleeding.

    c. PET (Positron Emission Tomography) Scan: PET scans can detect changes in brain metabolism and may be used to differentiate between different types of dementia, especially in the early stages.

6. Cerebrospinal Fluid Analysis:
   a. Lumbar Puncture: In some instances, a lumbar puncture may be performed to analyze cerebrospinal fluid for markers associated with Alzheimer's disease, such as beta-amyloid and tau proteins.
7. Functional Assessments:
   a. Activities of Daily Living (ADL) Assessment: This assesses an individual's ability to perform everyday tasks independently, such as dressing, grooming, and cooking.
   b. Instrumental Activities of Daily Living (IADL) Assessment evaluates more complex activities, including managing finances and medication.
8. Psychiatric Evaluation:
   a. Assessment of Mood and Behavior: A psychiatric evaluation helps identify symptoms of depression, anxiety, or behavioral changes, which are common in individuals with dementia.
9. Collaborative Approach:
   a. Multidisciplinary Team: Diagnosis often involves collaboration among healthcare professionals, including neurologists, geriatricians, psychiatrists, and neuropsychologists. Family members and caregivers play a crucial role in providing information about changes in behavior and cognitive function.

10. Follow-Up and Monitoring:
   a. Regular Monitoring: Dementia is a progressive condition, and frequent follow-up assessments help monitor changes in cognitive function, allowing for adjustments in care plans and interventions.

TREATMENT OF DEMENTIA

The treatment of dementia involves a comprehensive, multidisciplinary approach aimed at managing symptoms, enhancing quality of life, and providing support to both individuals with dementia and their caregivers. It's important to note that while there is no cure for most types of dementia, various interventions can help alleviate symptoms and improve overall well-being. The treatment plan is often individualized, taking into account the specific type of dementia, the stage of the condition, and the unique needs of the person affected. Here is an overview of the critical components of dementia treatment:

1. Medications:
    a. Cholinesterase Inhibitors: These medications, such as donepezil, rivastigmine, and galantamine, are commonly prescribed for Alzheimer's disease. They work by increasing levels of acetylcholine, a neurotransmitter involved in memory and learning.
    b. NMDA Receptor Antagonists: Memantine is an example of a medication that may be used to

manage symptoms in moderate to severe Alzheimer's disease. It works by regulating glutamate, another neurotransmitter involved in learning and memory.

2. Behavioral and Psychological Interventions:
   a. Cognitive Stimulation Therapy: Activities and exercises designed to stimulate cognitive function and engage individuals with dementia.
   b. Reality Orientation: Techniques to reinforce awareness of time, place, and person, helping individuals stay oriented to their surroundings.
   c. Reminiscence Therapy: Encouraging individuals to discuss and reflect on past experiences to improve mood and stimulate memory.

3. Occupational Therapy:
   a. Adaptive Strategies: Occupational therapists help individuals with dementia maintain independence by introducing adaptive strategies and tools for daily activities.
   b. Environmental Modifications: Creating a safe and supportive environment can enhance functioning and reduce confusion.

4. Physical Exercise:
   a. Regular Exercise Programs: Physical activity has been shown to have cognitive and emotional benefits for individuals with dementia. Exercise

can improve mood, reduce behavioral symptoms, and enhance overall well-being.

5. Nutritional Support:
    a. Balanced Diet: A nutritious and well-balanced diet is essential for overall health. Adequate nutrition supports physical and cognitive function.
    b. Supplements: In some cases, healthcare professionals may recommend supplements, such as vitamin B12 or omega-3 fatty acids, to support brain health.

6. Social Engagement:
    a. Social Activities: Maintaining social connections is vital for individuals with dementia. Participating in social activities and staying engaged with family and friends can improve mood and cognitive function.

7. Caregiver Support:
    a. Education and Training: Providing caregivers with information and training on managing and coping with the challenges of caring for someone with dementia.
    b. Respite Care: Offering caregivers regular breaks to rest and recharge is crucial for preventing caregiver burnout.

8. Symptom-Specific Approaches:
    a. Management of Agitation and Aggression: Strategies such as identifying triggers, maintaining

routines, and creating a calm environment can help manage behavioral symptoms.

b. Sleep Management: Establishing a consistent sleep routine and addressing factors contributing to sleep disturbances can improve overall well-being.

9. Clinical Trials and Research:

a. Participation in Research: In some cases, individuals with dementia may have the option to participate in clinical trials investigating new treatments or medications.

10. Advance Care Planning:

a. Discussion of Goals of Care: As dementia progresses, discussions about advance care planning, including preferences for end-of-life care, become essential to ensure that the individual's wishes are respected.

LIFESTYLE CHANGES

Lifestyle changes play a crucial role in the management of dementia, focusing on optimizing overall well-being, enhancing cognitive function, and providing support for individuals living with dementia and their caregivers. These changes encompass a variety of domains, including physical health, mental stimulation, social engagement, and environmental modifications. Here is an overview of lifestyle changes that can positively impact individuals with dementia:

1. Regular Physical Exercise:
   a. Benefits: Physical activity has been associated with numerous cognitive and emotional benefits for individuals with dementia. Regular exercise can improve mood, reduce behavioral symptoms, and enhance overall cognitive function.
   b. Activities: Tailored exercise programs, such as walking, chair exercises, and gentle stretching, promote physical health and contribute to a sense of well-being.
2. Brain-Healthy Diet:

a. Nutrient-rich foods: A balanced and nutritious diet supports overall health and brain function. Emphasizing fruits, vegetables, whole grains, and lean proteins can provide essential nutrients.

b. Hydration: Staying well-hydrated is crucial for cognitive function. Encouraging regular water intake is essential, as dehydration can negatively impact mood and cognition.

3. Cognitive Stimulation:

a. Engaging Activities: Activities that stimulate the mind, such as puzzles, games, and reading, can help maintain cognitive function. Cognitive stimulation therapy, involving structured activities, is often beneficial.

b. Memory Aids: Using memory aids such as calendars, notes, and electronic reminders can support individuals in daily tasks.

4. Social Engagement:

a. Maintaining Relationships: Maintaining social connections is vital for emotional well-being. Engaging in social activities, spending time with family and friends, and participating in community events can provide a sense of belonging.

b. Support Groups: Joining support groups for individuals with dementia and their caregivers offers an opportunity to share experiences, gain insights, and receive emotional support.

5. Sleep Hygiene:
   a. Establishing Routine: Maintaining a consistent sleep routine, including a regular bedtime and wake-up time, can improve sleep quality.
   b. Creating a Comfortable Environment: Ensuring a comfortable and calming sleep environment, with minimized disruptions and adequate lighting, contributes to better sleep.
6. Environmental Modifications:
   a. Safe and Supportive Spaces: Adapting the living environment to reduce hazards, enhance safety, and support independence is crucial. This may include removing tripping hazards, using labels and signs, and organizing spaces for easy navigation.
   b. Memory Aids in the Environment: Visual cues, such as color-coded labels or familiar objects, can assist in navigation and daily activities.
7. Stress Management:
   a. Relaxation Techniques: Incorporating relaxation techniques, such as deep breathing exercises, meditation, or mindfulness, can help manage stress and anxiety.
   b. Sensory Stimulation: Providing sensory stimulation, such as listening to music or enjoying nature, can have a calming effect.
8. Caregiver Support:

a. Education and Respite: Educating caregivers about dementia, its progression, and effective caregiving strategies is crucial. Offering respite care to caregivers allows for periodic breaks to prevent burnout.

b. Open Communication: Open and honest communication within the caregiving team fosters a supportive environment.

9. Routine and Predictability:

a. Establishing Routines: Maintaining daily routines and consistency in activities can provide a sense of predictability and security for individuals with dementia.

b. Minimizing Changes: Minimizing environmental or routine changes helps reduce confusion and anxiety.

10. Advance Care Planning:

a. Discussions About Future Care: As dementia progresses, discussions about advanced care planning become essential. Clarifying preferences for medical care, living arrangements, and end-of-life decisions ensures that the individual's wishes are known and respected.

CHAPTER TWO

The Role of Diet in Dementia

The role of diet in dementia has garnered significant attention as researchers explore the potential impact of nutritional choices on cognitive function and the risk of developing dementia. While no definitive diet can cure or prevent dementia, evidence suggests that specific dietary patterns may influence brain health and contribute to overall well-being. Here is a comprehensive overview of the role of diet in dementia:

1. Mediterranean Diet:
    a. Description: The Mediterranean diet, characterized by high consumption of fruits, vegetables, whole grains, fish, and healthy fats (e.g., olive oil), has been associated with a lower risk of cognitive decline and dementia.
    b. Rationale: Rich in antioxidants, omega-3 fatty acids, and anti-inflammatory compounds, the Mediterranean diet may contribute to neuroprotection and support cardiovascular health, which is linked to brain function.
2. Omega-3 Fatty Acids:
    a. Sources: Fatty fish (salmon, trout), walnuts, flaxseeds, and chia seeds are

rich in omega-3 fatty acids.
   b. Rationale: Omega-3 fatty acids are essential for brain health, particularly docosahexaenoic acid (DHA) and eicosapentaenoic acid (EPA). They play a role in maintaining the structure and function of brain cell membranes.
3. Antioxidant-Rich Foods:
   a. Sources: Berries, dark chocolate, leafy greens, and colorful vegetables are rich in antioxidants.
   b. Rationale: Antioxidants help neutralize free radicals, reducing oxidative stress that can contribute to cellular damage in the brain. High antioxidant intake may be associated with a lower risk of cognitive decline.
4. Vitamins and Minerals:
   a. Sources: Leafy greens, nuts, seeds, and fortified cereals are sources of vitamin E, B vitamins (including B12 and folate), and other essential minerals.
   b. Rationale: Adequate intake of vitamins and minerals is crucial for overall health, including brain function. Deficiencies in vitamin B12 and folate are linked to cognitive impairment.
5. Limiting Processed Foods and Sugar:
   a. Recommendation: Minimizing the intake of processed foods and added sugars is advisable.
   b. Rationale: A diet high in processed foods and sugars may contribute to

inflammation and negatively impact overall health, including brain health. It is linked to conditions such as insulin resistance and obesity, which are risk factors for dementia.

6. Moderate Alcohol Consumption:
   a. Recommendation: If alcohol is consumed, it should be done in moderation.
   b. Rationale: Excessive alcohol consumption is associated with an increased risk of dementia. Moderate alcohol intake, particularly of red wine, has been suggested to have potential cardiovascular benefits.

7. Hydration:
   a. Recommendation: Adequate hydration is essential for overall health, including cognitive function.
   b. Rationale: Dehydration can impair cognitive performance and exacerbate confusion. Maintaining proper hydration supports optimal brain function.

8. Individualized Approach:
   a. Consideration: Dietary recommendations should be individualized based on health status, existing conditions, and personal preferences.
   b. Rationale: Individuals may have varying nutritional needs and preferences, and a personalized approach ensures that

dietary changes are realistic and sustainable.

BENEFIT OF DEMENTIA DIET TO THE DEMENTIA PATIENT

A dementia diet, characterized by specific nutritional choices and dietary patterns, can offer several potential benefits to individuals living with dementia. While diet alone cannot cure or entirely prevent dementia, adopting a brain-healthy diet may positively impact cognitive function, overall health, and the quality of life for individuals facing this challenging condition. Here is an exploration of the benefits of a dementia diet:

1. Cognitive Support:
   a. Nutrient-Rich Foods: A diet rich in antioxidants, omega-3 fatty acids, and essential vitamins and minerals supports mental health. These nutrients play vital roles in brain function and may contribute to the preservation of cognitive abilities.
2. Reduced Oxidative Stress:
   a. Antioxidant Protection: Antioxidants found in fruits, vegetables, and dark-

colored berries help combat oxidative stress, which is implicated in the progression of dementia. Antioxidants neutralize free radicals, reducing cellular damage in the brain.

3. Heart Health Benefits:
   a. Mediterranean Diet Influence: Following a Mediterranean-style diet, which includes heart-healthy fats, lean proteins, and whole grains, can contribute to cardiovascular health. Cardiovascular health is closely linked to brain health, and reducing the risk of heart disease may have positive effects on cognitive function.

4. Inflammation Reduction:
   a. Omega-3 Fatty Acids: Foods rich in omega-3 fatty acids, such as fatty fish, walnuts, and flaxseeds, have anti-inflammatory properties. Chronic inflammation is associated with various chronic diseases affecting the brain.

5. Balanced Blood Sugar Levels:
   a. Whole Foods Emphasis: Prioritizing whole foods over processed and sugary options helps regulate blood sugar levels. Stable blood sugar levels are essential for preventing insulin resistance, which has been linked to cognitive decline.

6. Weight Management:
   a. Balanced Nutrient Intake: A well-balanced diet supports weight

management, reducing the risk of obesity. Obesity is associated with an increased risk of dementia, and maintaining a healthy weight contributes to overall well-being.

7. Improved Hydration:
   a. Adequate Fluid Intake: Staying adequately hydrated is crucial for cognitive function. Dehydration can lead to confusion fatigue, and exacerbate cognitive impairment. Encouraging adequate fluid intake supports optimal brain function.

8. Enhanced Mood and Behavior:
   a. Nutrient Influence on Neurotransmitters: Certain nutrients, such as those found in whole grains and lean proteins, play a role in producing neurotransmitters that influence mood. A well-nourished brain may contribute to better emotional well-being and behavior.

9. Support for Caregivers:
   a. Structured Meal Plans: Implementing structured meal plans that prioritize nutrient-dense foods can simplify meal preparation for caregivers. This may reduce stress and contribute to a more organized caregiving routine.

10. Potential Delay in Disease Progression:
    a. Overall Lifestyle Impact: While diet is just one component, adopting a brain-healthy diet as part of a comprehensive

lifestyle approach (including physical activity, mental stimulation, and social engagement) may contribute to a potential delay in the progression of cognitive decline.

FOODS TO INCLUDE

1. Fatty Fish:
   a. Examples: Salmon, mackerel, trout.
   b. Reason: Rich in omega-3 fatty acids, particularly DHA, which supports brain health and may have cognitive benefits.
2. Colorful Fruits and Vegetables:
   a. Examples: Berries, leafy greens, broccoli, sweet potatoes.
   b. Reason: High in antioxidants and vitamins that combat oxidative stress and support overall health.
3. Whole Grains:
   a. Examples: Quinoa, brown rice, whole wheat.
   b. Reason: Provide sustained energy, fiber, and essential nutrients for brain function.
4. Nuts and Seeds:
   a. Examples: Walnuts, almonds, flaxseeds, and chia seeds.
   b. Reason: Good omega-3 fatty acids, antioxidants, and vitamin E sources.
5. Lean Proteins:
   a. Examples: Chicken, turkey, beans, and lentils.
   b. Reason: It is essential for muscle health

and provides a source of amino acids critical for neurotransmitter function.

6. Healthy Fats:
   a. Examples: Olive oil avocados.
   b. Reason: Provide monounsaturated fats, which support cardiovascular health and may benefit the brain.
7. Low-Fat Dairy or Dairy Alternatives:
   a. Examples: Greek yogurt and almond milk.
   b. Reason: Good sources of calcium and vitamin D for bone health.
8. Herbs and Spices:
   a. Examples: Turmeric, cinnamon, rosemary.
   b. Reason: Some herbs and spices have anti-inflammatory properties and antioxidants.
9. Hydration:
   a. Water, Herbal Teas.
   b. Reason: Maintaining proper hydration is crucial for cognitive function and overall well-being.
10. Dark Chocolate:
    a. Reason: In moderation, dark chocolate with high cocoa content provides antioxidants and may have mood-enhancing benefits.

FOODS TO LIMIT OR AVOID

1. Processed Foods:
    a. Examples: Fast food pre-packaged snacks.
    b. Reason: Often high in unhealthy fats, sugars, and additives, which can contribute to inflammation.
2. Sugary Foods and Beverages:
    a. Examples: Sodas, candies, and pastries.
    b. Reason: Excessive sugar intake may contribute to inflammation and negatively impact overall health.
3. Saturated and Trans Fats:
    a. Sources: Fried foods, processed meats.
    b. Reason: High intake may contribute to cardiovascular issues, negatively impacting brain health.
4. Excessive Red Meat:
    a. Reason: While lean meats are beneficial, excessive red meat consumption may be linked to specific health issues.
5. High-Sodium Foods:
    a. Examples: Processed foods salty snacks.
    b. Reason: High sodium intake can contribute to hypertension and

negatively impact cardiovascular health.

6. Alcohol:
   a. Reason: Excessive alcohol consumption is associated with an increased risk of dementia. If consumed, it should be in moderation.
7. Caffeine:
   a. Reason: While moderate caffeine intake is generally considered safe, excessive consumption may impact sleep, leading to cognitive issues.
8. Unhealthy Cooking Oils:
   a. Examples: Vegetable oils high in omega-6 fatty acids.
   b. Reason: An imbalance between omega-3 and omega-6 fatty acids may contribute to inflammation.
9. Artificial Additives:
   a. Examples: Artificial sweeteners and preservatives.
   b. Reason: Some individuals may be sensitive to artificial additives, and their impact on health is still under research.
10. Highly Processed or High-Glycemic Carbohydrates:
    a. Examples: White bread sugary cereals.
    b. Reason: It may lead to rapid spikes and crashes in blood sugar levels.

SAMPLE MEAL PLAN

Creating a meal plan for individuals with dementia involves careful consideration of nutritional needs, preferences, and practicality. A well-balanced and varied diet is essential to provide nutrients, support cognitive function, and maintain overall health. Here's a sample meal plan for seven days, incorporating a mix of nutrient-dense foods while considering the challenges that individuals with dementia may face:

Day 1:

Breakfast:

• Oatmeal with mixed berries and a sprinkle of walnuts.

• Greek yogurt with honey and a side of sliced banana.

Mid-Morning Snack:

• Apple slices with almond butter.

Lunch:

• Grilled chicken salad with mixed greens, cherry tomatoes, cucumbers, and a vinaigrette dressing.

• Quinoa or brown rice on the side.

Afternoon Snack:

• Carrot and cucumber sticks with hummus.

Dinner:

• Baked salmon with a lemon and herb marinade.

• Roasted sweet potatoes and steamed broccoli.

• Whole grain roll on the side.

Evening Snack:

• A small bowl of mixed berries.

Day 2:

Breakfast:

• Whole grain toast with avocado and poached eggs.

• Orange slices on the side.

Mid-Morning Snack:

• Greek yogurt parfait with layers of granola and fresh berries.

Lunch:

• Lentil soup with a side of whole grain crackers.

• Spinach and strawberry salad with balsamic vinaigrette.

Afternoon Snack:

• Handful of mixed nuts (walnuts, almonds, and cashews).

Dinner:

• Stir-fried tofu with mixed vegetables (bell peppers, broccoli, snap peas).

• Brown rice or quinoa.

Evening Snack:

• Sliced peaches with a dollop of cottage cheese.

Day 3:

Breakfast:

• Smoothie with spinach, banana, berries, and almond milk.

• Whole grain toast with peanut butter.

Mid-Morning Snack:

• Cottage cheese with pineapple chunks.

Lunch:

• Turkey and vegetable wrap with whole grain tortilla.

• Mixed green salad with a light dressing.

Afternoon Snack:

• Celery sticks with cream cheese.

Dinner:

• Grilled shrimp skewers with a side of quinoa.

• Steamed asparagus and a small baked potato.

Evening Snack:

• A small bowl of mixed melon.

Day 4:

Breakfast:

• Scrambled eggs with spinach and feta cheese.

• Whole grain toast with jam.

• Sliced melon on the side.

Mid-Morning Snack:

• A smoothie with mixed berries, bananas, and yogurt.

Lunch:

• Chicken and vegetable stir-fry with brown rice.

- Mixed fruit salad with a drizzle of honey.

Afternoon Snack:

- Whole grain crackers with cheese slices.

Dinner:

- Baked cod with a lemon-dill sauce.
- Mashed sweet potatoes and green beans.
- Whole grain roll.

Evening Snack:

- Greek yogurt with a sprinkle of granola.

Day 5:

Breakfast:

- Cottage cheese pancakes with fresh strawberries.
- Orange juice on the side.

Mid-Morning Snack:

- Sliced cucumber with tzatziki dip.

Lunch:

- Quinoa salad with chickpeas, cherry tomatoes, and feta cheese.
- Grilled chicken skewers.

Afternoon Snack:

- Apple slices with a small portion of cheese.

Dinner:

- Beef and vegetable stew with whole grain barley.
- Steamed broccoli and carrots.

Evening Snack:

• Trail mix with dried fruits and mixed nuts.

Day 6:

Breakfast:

• Yogurt parfait with layers of granola, sliced bananas, and a drizzle of honey.

• Whole grain toast with almond butter.

Mid-Morning Snack:

• Cherry tomatoes with mozzarella cheese.

Lunch:

• Lentil and vegetable soup.

• Turkey and avocado wrap with a side of mixed greens.

Afternoon Snack:

• Sliced bell peppers with hummus.

Dinner:

• Baked chicken with rosemary and garlic.

• Quinoa pilaf with mixed vegetables.

• Steamed asparagus.

Evening Snack:

• Sliced mango with a dollop of Greek yogurt.

Day 7:

Breakfast:

• Whole grain bagel with smoked salmon, cream cheese, and capers.

• Fresh fruit salad.

Mid-Morning Snack:

- Banana slices with a smear of almond butter.

Lunch:

- Shrimp and avocado salad with a citrus vinaigrette.
- Quinoa or brown rice on the side.

Afternoon Snack:

- Trail mix with a mix of nuts and dried fruits.

Dinner:

- Vegetable and tofu curry with basmati rice.
- Steamed green beans.

Evening Snack:

- A small bowl of mixed berries with a sprinkle of shredded coconut.

CHAPTER THREE

Nutrient-Rich Foods Recipes
Grilled Salmon with Lemon and Dill

Meal Description:

This Grilled Salmon with Lemon and Dill recipe offers a delightful combination of flavors, featuring succulent salmon infused with zesty lemon and aromatic dill. It's a light and nutritious meal that's easy to prepare, perfect for a quick and healthy dinner.

Ingredients:

- Four salmon fillets (6 ounces each)
- Two tablespoons fresh dill, chopped
- Two tablespoons extra-virgin olive oil
- Two tablespoons of fresh lemon juice
- Two teaspoons of lemon zest
- Two cloves garlic, minced
- Salt and black pepper to taste
- Lemon wedges for serving

Instructions:

1. Prepare the Marinade:
   a. Whisk together the chopped dill, olive oil, lemon juice, lemon zest, minced garlic, salt, and black pepper in a small bowl.
2. Marinate the Salmon:
   a. Place the salmon fillets in a shallow dish or a resealable plastic bag. Pour the marinade over the salmon, ensuring it's evenly coated. Marinate in the

refrigerator for at least 30 minutes, allowing the flavors to meld.

3. Preheat the Grill:
   a. Preheat your grill to medium-high heat. Brush the grates with oil to prevent sticking.
4. Grill the Salmon:
   a. Remove the salmon from the marinade, letting any excess drip off. Place the fillets on the preheated grill. Grill for approximately 4-5 minutes per side or until the salmon is cooked through and quickly flakes with a fork.
5. Serve:
   a. Transfer the grilled salmon to a serving platter. Garnish with additional fresh dill and lemon wedges for squeezing over the top.
6. Enjoy:
   a. Serve the Grilled Salmon with Lemon and Dill alongside your favorite sides such as steamed vegetables, quinoa, or a light salad.

Nutrition Information (Per Serving):

- Calories: 220

- Protein: 28g

- Fat: 11g

- Saturated Fat: 2g

- Carbohydrates: 2g

- Fiber: 0.5g

- Sugars: 0.5g
- Cholesterol: 75mg
- Sodium: 120mg

QUINOA AND BLACK BEAN SALAD WITH AVOCADO

Meal Description:

This Quinoa and Black Bean Salad with Avocado is a vibrant and nutritious dish that combines the goodness of protein-rich quinoa, fiber-packed black beans, and creamy avocado. It's a refreshing salad with a zesty lime dressing, perfect for a light lunch or a flavorful side dish.

Ingredients:

For the Salad:

- 1 cup quinoa, cooked and cooled
- One can (15 oz) black beans, drained and rinsed
- 1 cup cherry tomatoes, halved
- 1 cup cucumber, diced
- 1/2 cup red bell pepper, diced
- 1/4 cup red onion, finely chopped
- 1/4 cup fresh cilantro, chopped

For the Dressing:

- Three tablespoons extra-virgin olive oil

- Two tablespoons of fresh lime juice
- One teaspoon of ground cumin
- One teaspoon of chili powder
- Salt and black pepper to taste

Additional:

- One ripe avocado, diced (added just before serving)

Instructions:

1. Prepare Quinoa:
   a. Cook quinoa according to package instructions. Once cooked, let it cool to room temperature.
2. Assemble Salad:
   a. Combine the cooked quinoa, black beans, cherry tomatoes, cucumber, red bell pepper, red onion, and fresh cilantro in a large mixing bowl.
3. Prepare Dressing:
   a. Whisk together the olive oil, lime juice, ground cumin, chili powder, salt, and black pepper in a small bowl to create the dressing.
4. Dress the Salad:
   a. Pour the dressing over the salad and toss gently until all ingredients are well coated.
5. Chill:
   a. Refrigerate the salad for at least 30 minutes to allow the flavors to meld.
6. Add Avocado:
   a. Just before serving, gently fold in the diced avocado to preserve its freshness

and creaminess.
7. Serve:
   a. Spoon the Quinoa and Black Bean Salad with Avocado onto a serving platter or individual plates.
8. Enjoy:
   a. Serve as a standalone salad or as a side dish with grilled chicken or fish. Garnish with extra cilantro if desired.

Nutrition Information (Per Serving):

- Calories: 320

- Protein: 10g

- Fat: 16g

- Saturated Fat: 2g

- Carbohydrates: 38g

- Fiber: 9g

- Sugars: 2g

- Cholesterol: 0mg

- Sodium: 180mg

BAKED CHICKEN BREAST WITH SWEET POTATOES AND BROCCOLI

Meal Description:

This Baked Chicken Breast with Sweet Potatoes and Broccoli is a wholesome and well-balanced dish that brings together lean protein, complex carbohydrates, and nutrient-rich vegetables. With a hint of savory and sweet flavors, it's an easy-to-make, one-pan meal perfect for a nourishing dinner.

Ingredients:

For the Chicken:

- Four boneless, skinless chicken breasts
- Two tablespoons of olive oil
- Two teaspoons of garlic powder
- Two teaspoons paprika
- One teaspoon of dried thyme
- Salt and black pepper to taste

For the Vegetables:

- Two large sweet potatoes, peeled and cubed
- 3 cups broccoli florets
- Two tablespoons of olive oil
- One teaspoon of garlic powder
- Salt and black pepper to taste

Instructions:

1. Preheat the Oven:
   a. Preheat the oven to 400°F (200°C).
2. Prepare the Chicken:
   a. Mix the garlic powder, paprika, dried thyme, salt, and black pepper in a small bowl. Brush each chicken breast with olive oil, then season both sides with the spice mixture.
3. Prepare the Vegetables:
   a. Toss the sweet potato cubes and broccoli florets in a separate bowl with olive oil, garlic powder, salt, and black pepper until evenly coated.
4. Assemble on a Baking Sheet:
   a. Place the seasoned chicken breasts on one side of a large baking sheet and the seasoned sweet potatoes and broccoli on the other side. Ensure a single layer for even cooking.
5. Bake:
   a. Bake in the preheated oven for approximately 25-30 minutes or until the chicken reaches an internal temperature of 165°F (74°C) and the vegetables are tender. Cooking times

may vary based on the thickness of the chicken breasts.

6. Rest and Serve:
    a. Allow the chicken to rest for a few minutes before slicing. Serve the shredded chicken over a bed of sweet potatoes and broccoli.
7. Enjoy:
    a. Enjoy this wholesome Baked Chicken Breast with Sweet Potatoes and Broccoli as a complete and satisfying meal.

Nutrition Information (Per Serving):

- Calories: 380
- Protein: 30g
- Fat: 14g
- Saturated Fat: 2.5g
- Carbohydrates: 35g
- Fiber: 7g
- Sugars: 7g
- Cholesterol: 75mg
- Sodium: 150mg

LENTIL SOUP WITH SPINACH AND TOMATOES

Meal Description:

This Lentil Soup with Spinach and Tomatoes is a hearty and nutritious dish combining protein-rich lentils and vibrant vegetables. Packed with flavors from aromatic herbs and tomatoes, this soup is delicious and an excellent source of fiber and essential nutrients.

Ingredients:

- 1 cup dried green or brown lentils, rinsed and drained
- One tablespoon of olive oil
- One onion, finely chopped
- Two carrots diced
- Two celery stalks, diced
- Three cloves garlic, minced
- One teaspoon of ground cumin
- One teaspoon of ground coriander
- One teaspoon of smoked paprika
- One can (14 oz) diced tomatoes, undrained

- 6 cups vegetable or chicken broth
- 2 cups fresh spinach, chopped
- Salt and black pepper to taste
- Fresh lemon wedges for Serving (optional)

Instructions:

1. Prepare Lentils:
   a. Rinse the lentils under cold water and set aside.
2. Sauté Vegetables:
   a. In a large pot, heat olive oil over medium heat. Add chopped onion, diced carrots, and diced celery. Sauté until the vegetables are softened, about 5-7 minutes.
3. Add Aromatics:
   a. Stir in minced garlic, ground cumin, ground coriander, and smoked paprika. Cook for an additional 1-2 minutes until fragrant.
4. Combine Lentils and Tomatoes:
   a. Add the rinsed lentils, diced tomatoes (with their juices), and broth to the pot. Bring the mixture to a boil.
5. Simmer:
   a. Reduce the heat to low, cover the pot, and let the soup simmer for about 25-30 minutes or until the lentils are tender.
6. Add Spinach:
   a. Stir in the chopped spinach and cook for an additional 5 minutes or until the spinach is wilted.

7. Season:
    a. Season the soup with salt and black pepper to taste. Adjust the seasoning as needed.
8. Serve:
    a. Ladle the Lentil Soup with Spinach and Tomatoes into bowls. Optionally, squeeze fresh lemon juice over each Serving for a burst of citrus flavor.
9. Enjoy:
    a. Enjoy this wholesome and flavorful lentil soup as a comforting meal. Serve with crusty bread or a side salad if desired.

Nutrition Information (Per Serving):

• Calories: 220

• Protein: 12g

• Fat: 4g

• Saturated Fat: 0.5g

• Carbohydrates: 38g

• Fiber: 14g

• Sugars: 6g

• Cholesterol: 0mg

• Sodium: 800mg

GREEK YOGURT PARFAIT WITH FRESH BERRIES AND ALMONDS

Meal Description:

This Greek Yogurt Parfait with Fresh Berries and Almonds is a delightful and nutritious treat, combining the creaminess of Greek yogurt with the sweetness of fresh berries and the crunch of almonds. Whether enjoyed as a satisfying breakfast, a wholesome snack, or a light dessert, this parfait is a burst of flavors and textures.

Ingredients:

• 1 cup Greek yogurt (unsweetened)

• One tablespoon of honey or maple syrup (optional for sweetness)

• 1 cup mixed fresh berries (strawberries, blueberries, raspberries)

• Two tablespoons sliced almonds

• 1/2 teaspoon vanilla extract (optional)

• Fresh mint leaves for garnish (optional)

Instructions:

1. Prepare Greek Yogurt:
   a. Mix Greek yogurt with honey or maple syrup (if using) and vanilla extract in a bowl. Adjust sweetness to taste.
2. Layering the Parfait:
   a. Start by spooning a layer of the sweetened Greek yogurt into serving glasses or bowls.
3. Add Fresh Berries:
   a. Top the yogurt layer with a generous portion of mixed fresh berries. Ensure an even distribution of different berries for variety.
4. Repeat Layers:
   a. Repeat the layering process by adding another layer of sweetened Greek yogurt on top of the berries.
5. Top with Almonds:
   a. Sprinkle sliced almonds on the top layer for a delightful crunch and added protein.
6. Garnish (Optional):
   a. Garnish the parfait with fresh mint leaves for a touch of freshness and visual appeal.
7. Serve Immediately:
   a. Serve the Greek Yogurt Parfait with Fresh Berries and Almonds immediately, allowing the layers to meld for a harmonious combination of flavors.
8. Enjoy:

      a. Enjoy this wholesome and satisfying parfait as a delicious and nutrient-packed treat.

Nutrition Information (Per Serving):

- Calories: 250
- Protein: 18g
- Fat: 10g
- Saturated Fat: 1g
- Carbohydrates: 25g
- Fiber: 5g
- Sugars: 16g
- Cholesterol: 10mg
- Sodium: 50mg

TURKEY AND VEGETABLE STIR-FRY

Meal Description:

This Turkey and Vegetable Stir-Fry is a quick and flavorful dish that combines lean ground turkey with a colorful array of vegetables, creating a nutritious and satisfying meal. The stir-fry is seasoned with a savory sauce, making it a delicious and well-balanced option for lunch or dinner.

Ingredients:

For the Stir-Fry:

- 1 lb ground turkey (lean)
- Two tablespoons soy sauce (low sodium)
- One tablespoon of hoisin sauce
- One tablespoon of oyster sauce
- One tablespoon of sesame oil
- Two tablespoons of vegetable oil
- Three cloves garlic, minced
- One tablespoon of fresh ginger, grated

- One red bell pepper, thinly sliced
- One yellow bell pepper, thinly sliced
- 1 medium carrot, julienned
- 1 cup snap peas, ends trimmed
- 1 cup broccoli florets
- Four green onions, sliced (for garnish)
- Sesame seeds for garnish (optional)

For Serving:

- Cooked brown rice or quinoa

Instructions:

1. Prepare Sauce:
   a. Whisk together soy sauce, hoisin sauce, and oyster sauce in a small bowl. Set aside.
2. Cook Ground Turkey:
   a. Heat one tablespoon of vegetable oil over medium-high heat in a wok or large skillet. Add ground turkey, cook until browned, and break it apart with a spatula. Once cooked, transfer the turkey to a plate.
3. Sauté Aromatics and Vegetables:
   a. In the same pan, add the remaining tablespoon of vegetable oil. Sauté minced garlic and grated ginger until fragrant. Add sliced bell peppers, julienned carrots, snap peas, and broccoli florets. Stir-fry for 3-5 minutes or until the vegetables are crisp-tender.
4. Combine Turkey and Vegetables:

a. Return the cooked turkey to the pan with the vegetables. Mix well to combine.

5. Add Sauce:

   a. Pour the prepared sauce over the turkey and vegetables. Stir to coat evenly and allow the sauce to thicken slightly.

6. Finish with Sesame Oil:

   a. Drizzle sesame oil over the stir-fry and toss to combine. This adds a rich and nutty flavor to the dish.

7. Serve:

   a. Serve the Turkey and Vegetable Stir-Fry over cooked brown rice or quinoa.

8. Garnish and Enjoy:

   a. Garnish with sliced green onions and sesame seeds if desired. Serve immediately and enjoy this delicious and wholesome stir-fry.

Nutrition Information (Per Serving, excluding rice/quinoa):

- Calories: 300
- Protein: 25g
- Fat: 18g
- Saturated Fat: 4g
- Carbohydrates: 15g
- Fiber: 4g
- Sugars: 6g
- Cholesterol: 70mg
- Sodium: 700mg

SPINACH AND FETA STUFFED CHICKEN BREAST

Meal Description:

This Spinach and Feta Stuffed Chicken Breast is a flavorful and elegant dish that combines tender chicken breast with a rich and savory spinach and feta filling. Baked to perfection, this dish is delicious and provides a delightful burst of Mediterranean flavors.

Ingredients:

For the Stuffed Chicken Breast:

- Four boneless, skinless chicken breasts
- 2 cups fresh spinach, chopped
- 1 cup feta cheese, crumbled
- 1/4 cup sun-dried tomatoes, chopped
- Two cloves garlic, minced
- One tablespoon of olive oil
- One teaspoon dried oregano
- Salt and black pepper to taste

For Seasoning the Chicken:

- Two tablespoons of olive oil
- One teaspoon of dried thyme
- One teaspoon of dried rosemary
- Salt and black pepper to taste

Instructions:

1. Preheat the Oven:
    a. Preheat the oven to 375°F (190°C).
2. Prepare the Spinach and Feta Filling:
    a. In a pan, heat one tablespoon of olive oil over medium heat. Add minced garlic and cook until fragrant. Add chopped spinach and cook until wilted. Remove from heat and let it cool.
    b. Combine the cooked spinach, crumbled feta cheese, chopped sun-dried tomatoes, dried oregano, salt, and black pepper in a bowl. Mix well to create the stuffing.
3. Prepare Chicken Breasts:
    a. On a clean surface, lay out the chicken breasts. Using a sharp knife, make a horizontal slit in each chicken breast to create a pocket without cutting all the way through.
4. Stuff the Chicken:
    a. Stuff each chicken breast with the spinach and feta mixture, distributing it evenly among the breasts.
5. Season and Sear:
    a. Mix olive oil, dried thyme, rosemary, salt, and black pepper in a small bowl.

Rub this mixture over the outside of each chicken breast.

b. In an oven-safe skillet, heat olive oil over medium-high heat. Sear the stuffed chicken breasts for 2-3 minutes on each side until golden brown.

6. Bake:

a. Transfer the skillet to the preheated oven. Bake for 20-25 minutes or until the chicken reaches an internal temperature of 165°F (74°C) and is no longer pink in the center.

7. Rest and Serve:

a. Allow the Spinach and Feta Stuffed Chicken Breast to rest for a few minutes before slicing.

8. Serve:

a. Serve the stuffed chicken breasts on a platter, and spoon any pan juices over the top.

9. Enjoy:

a. Enjoy this elegant and flavorful dish with your favorite sides, such as roasted vegetables or a fresh salad.

Nutrition Information (Per Serving):

• Calories: 380

• Protein: 40g

• Fat: 20g

• Saturated Fat: 8g

• Carbohydrates: 8g

• Fiber: 3g

- Sugars: 3g
- Cholesterol: 120mg
- Sodium: 700mg

ROASTED BRUSSELS SPROUTS WITH POMEGRANATE SEEDS

Meal Description:

This Roasted Brussels Sprouts with Pomegranate Seeds dish is a festive and flavorful side that combines the nutty taste of roasted Brussels sprouts with the sweet and tart burst of pomegranate seeds. It's a colorful and nutritious addition to any meal, especially during the holiday season.

Ingredients:

• 1 lb Brussels sprouts, trimmed and halved

• Two tablespoons of olive oil

• Salt and black pepper to taste

• 1/4 cup pomegranate seeds

• Two tablespoons of balsamic glaze (or balsamic reduction)

Instructions:

1. Preheat the Oven:
   a. Preheat the oven to 400°F (200°C).
2. Prepare Brussels Sprouts:
   a. Trim the ends of the Brussels sprouts and cut them in half.
3. Coat with Olive Oil:
   a. Toss the Brussels sprouts with olive oil in a large mixing bowl, ensuring they are evenly coated.
4. Season:
   a. Season the Brussels sprouts with salt and black pepper according to taste. Toss again to distribute the seasoning.
5. Roast:
   a. Spread the Brussels sprouts in a single layer on a baking sheet. Roast in the preheated oven for 20-25 minutes or until the sprouts are golden brown and crispy at the edges.
6. Add Pomegranate Seeds:
   a. Remove the roasted Brussels sprouts from the oven and transfer them to a serving dish. Sprinkle the pomegranate seeds over the top.
7. Drizzle with Balsamic Glaze:
   a. Drizzle the balsamic glaze or reduction over the Brussels sprouts and pomegranate seeds. The sweet and tangy glaze adds depth of flavor.
8. Serve:
   a. Serve the Roasted Brussels Sprouts with Pomegranate Seeds immediately,

allowing the vibrant colors and flavors to shine.

9. Enjoy:

• Enjoy this festive and nutritious side dish alongside your favorite main courses, such as roast chicken or grilled salmon.

Nutrition Information (Per Serving):

• Calories: 120

• Protein: 4g

• Fat: 7g

• Saturated Fat: 1g

• Carbohydrates: 14g

• Fiber: 4g

• Sugars: 6g

• Cholesterol: 0mg

• Sodium: 20mg

CHICKPEA AND VEGETABLE CURRY

Meal Description:

This Chickpea and Vegetable Curry is a delicious and hearty plant-based dish that brings together the rich flavors of chickpeas, colorful vegetables, and aromatic spices. Perfectly balanced, it's a satisfying meal that's easy to prepare and packed with nutrients.

Ingredients:

For the Curry:

- Two tablespoons of vegetable oil
- One large onion, finely chopped
- Three cloves garlic, minced
- One tablespoon of fresh ginger, grated
- One tablespoon of curry powder
- One teaspoon of ground cumin
- One teaspoon of ground coriander
- 1/2 teaspoon turmeric
- 1/2 teaspoon chili powder (adjust to taste)
- One can (15 oz) chickpeas, drained and rinsed
- One can (14 oz) diced tomatoes, undrained

- 1 cup coconut milk
- Salt and black pepper to taste

Vegetables (Choose a mix of your favorites):

- 1 cup cauliflower florets
- 1 cup carrot, sliced
- 1 cup bell peppers, diced
- 1 cup baby spinach leaves
- 1 cup peas (fresh or frozen)

For Serving:

- Cooked basmati rice or naan bread

Instructions:

1. Sauté Aromatics:
   a. Heat vegetable oil over medium heat in a large pot or deep skillet. Add finely chopped onions and sauté until translucent.
2. Add Spices:
   a. Stir in minced garlic and grated ginger. Add curry powder, cumin, coriander, turmeric, and chili powder. Sauté for 1-2 minutes until the spices are fragrant.
3. Combine Chickpeas and Tomatoes:
   a. Add chickpeas, diced tomatoes (with their juices), and coconut milk to the pot. Stir well to combine.
4. Bring to a Simmer:
   a. Bring the mixture to a simmer and let it cook for 10 minutes, allowing the flavors to meld.

5. Add Vegetables:
    a. Add the selected vegetables to the pot. If using cauliflower and carrots, add them first, as they take longer to cook. Simmer until the vegetables are tender but still vibrant.
6. Season:
    a. Season the curry with salt and black pepper to taste. Adjust the seasoning as needed.
7. Finish with Spinach and Peas:
    a. Add baby spinach leaves and peas to the pot. Cook until the spinach is wilted and the peas are heated through.
8. Serve:
    a. Serve the Chickpea and Vegetable Curry over cooked basmati rice or with naan bread.
9. Enjoy:
    a. Enjoy this flavorful and nutritious curry as a satisfying plant-based meal.

Nutrition Information (Per Serving, excluding rice/naan):

• Calories: 320

• Protein: 9g

• Fat: 18g

• Saturated Fat: 12g

• Carbohydrates: 33g

• Fiber: 9g

• Sugars: 7g

- Cholesterol: 0mg
- Sodium: 680mg

SHRIMP AND ASPARAGUS STIR-FRY

Meal Description:

This Shrimp and Asparagus Stir-Fry is a quick and flavorful dish showcasing shrimp's succulence paired with crisp asparagus and a savory sauce. It's a light and nutritious stir-fry perfect for a speedy weeknight dinner.

Ingredients:

For the Stir-Fry:

- 1 lb large shrimp, peeled and deveined
- One bunch of asparagus, trimmed and cut into bite-sized pieces
- Two tablespoons of vegetable oil
- Three cloves garlic, minced
- One tablespoon of fresh ginger, grated
- One red bell pepper, thinly sliced
- Two tablespoons soy sauce (low sodium)
- One tablespoon of oyster sauce
- One teaspoon of sesame oil

- One tablespoon of rice vinegar

- One teaspoon of cornstarch mixed with two tablespoons water (optional for thickening)

For Serving:

- Cooked brown rice or noodles

Instructions:

1. Prepare Shrimp:
   a. If you still need to do so, peel and devein the shrimp. Pat them dry with paper towels.
2. Sauté Shrimp:
   a. In a wok or large skillet, heat vegetable oil over medium-high heat. Add minced garlic and grated ginger. Sauté for about 30 seconds until fragrant.
   b. Add shrimp to the wok and cook for 2-3 minutes per side or until they turn pink and opaque. Remove the shrimp from the wok and set aside.
3. Cook Asparagus and Bell Pepper:
   a. In the same wok, add a bit more oil if needed. Add asparagus and sliced red bell pepper. Stir-fry for 3-4 minutes or until the vegetables are crisp-tender.
4. Combine Shrimp and Vegetables:
   a. Return the cooked shrimp to the wok with the vegetables. Toss to combine.
5. Prepare Sauce:
   a. Whisk together soy sauce, oyster sauce, sesame oil, and rice vinegar in a small bowl. Pour the sauce over the shrimp

and vegetables.

6. Thicken Sauce (Optional):
   a. If desired, mix cornstarch with water to create a slurry. Add it to the wok to thicken the sauce. Stir well.
7. Serve:
   a. Serve the Shrimp and Asparagus Stir-Fry over cooked brown rice or noodles.
8. Enjoy:
   a. Enjoy this delicious and quick stir-fry as a wholesome meal with a perfect balance of flavors.

Nutrition Information (Per Serving, excluding rice/noodles):

• Calories: 280

• Protein: 30g

• Fat: 12g

• Saturated Fat: 1.5g

• Carbohydrates: 15g

• Fiber: 5g

• Sugars: 4g

• Cholesterol: 220mg

• Sodium: 700mg

CHAPTER FOUR

Omega-3 Fatty Acids Recipes
Walnut-Crusted Baked Cod

Meal Description:

This Walnut-Crusted Baked Cod is a delicious and nutritious dish that features tender cod fillets coated in a crunchy walnut crust. Baking the cod preserves its natural flavor while the walnut coating adds a delightful texture and nutty taste. This recipe is easy to make and provides a healthy option for a satisfying dinner.

Ingredients:

For the Walnut Crust:

- 1 cup walnuts, finely chopped
- 1/2 cup breadcrumbs (whole wheat or panko)
- One teaspoon of dried thyme
- One teaspoon of dried parsley
- 1/2 teaspoon garlic powder
- Salt and black pepper to taste

For the Cod:

- Four cod fillets (about 6 ounces each)
- Two tablespoons of Dijon mustard
- One tablespoon of olive oil
- Lemon wedges for serving

Instructions:

1. Preheat the Oven:
   a. Preheat the oven to 400°F (200°C). Line a baking sheet with parchment paper or

lightly grease it.
2. Prepare Walnut Crust:
   a. In a bowl, combine finely chopped walnuts, breadcrumbs, dried thyme, parsley, garlic powder, salt, and black pepper. Mix well to create the walnut crust mixture.
3. Coat Cod Fillets:
   a. Brush each cod fillet with Dijon mustard, ensuring an even coating on both sides.
4. Apply Walnut Crust:
   a. Press the mustard-coated cod fillets into the walnut crust mixture, ensuring that the crust adheres to the fish.
5. Place on Baking Sheet:
   a. Place the coated cod fillets on the prepared baking sheet.
6. Drizzle with Olive Oil:
   a. Drizzle olive oil over the top of each cod fillet. This adds moisture and helps the crust to brown nicely.
7. Bake:
   a. Bake in the preheated oven for 15-20 minutes or until the cod is cooked through and the walnut crust is golden brown and crispy.
8. Serve:
   a. Transfer the Walnut-Crusted Baked Cod to serving plates. Serve with lemon wedges on the side for a fresh burst of citrus flavor.
9. Enjoy:

a. Enjoy this delightful and wholesome dish alongside your favorite sides, such as roasted vegetables or a quinoa salad.

Nutrition Information (Per Serving):

- Calories: 350
- Protein: 30g
- Fat: 23g
- Saturated Fat: 2g
- Carbohydrates: 10g
- Fiber: 3g
- Sugars: 1g
- Cholesterol: 60mg
- Sodium: 300mg

CHIA SEED PUDDING WITH BERRIES

Meal Description:

This Chia Seed Pudding with Berries is a delightful and nutritious treat that can be enjoyed for breakfast, as a snack, or even as a healthy dessert. When mixed with liquid, the chia seeds create a pudding-like consistency, and topping it with a medley of fresh berries adds flavor and additional nutrients.

Ingredients:

For the Chia Seed Pudding:

• 1/4 cup chia seeds

• 1 cup almond milk (or any milk of your choice)

• One tablespoon of honey or maple syrup (optional for sweetness)

• 1/2 teaspoon vanilla extract (optional)

For Topping:

• 1 cup mixed berries (strawberries, blueberries, raspberries)

• Fresh mint leaves for garnish (optional)

Instructions:

1. Prepare Chia Seed Pudding:
   a. In a bowl, combine chia seeds, almond milk, honey or maple syrup (if using), and vanilla extract. Stir well to ensure the chia seeds are evenly distributed.
2. Let it Set:
   a. Cover the bowl and refrigerate the mixture for at least 2 hours or overnight. The chia seeds will absorb the liquid and create a pudding-like texture.
3. Stir Before Serving:
   a. Before serving, give the chia seed pudding a good stir to break up any clumps and ensure a smooth consistency.
4. Assemble with Berries:
   a. Spoon the chia seed pudding into serving glasses or bowls. Top with a generous portion of mixed berries.
5. Garnish (Optional):
   a. Garnish the Chia Seed Pudding with Berries with fresh mint leaves for a touch of freshness and visual appeal.
6. Serve:
   a. Serve immediately and enjoy this wholesome and satisfying chia seed pudding.
7. Variations:
   a. Customize your pudding by adding sliced bananas, chopped nuts, or a dollop of Greek yogurt.

8. Enjoy:

a. Whether enjoyed as a nutritious breakfast or a guilt-free dessert, this Chia Seed Pudding with Berries is a tasty and healthful option.

Nutrition Information (Per Serving):

- Calories: 220
- Protein: 5g
- Fat: 10g
- Saturated Fat: 1g
- Carbohydrates: 30g
- Fiber: 12g
- Sugars: 12g
- Cholesterol: 0mg
- Sodium: 100mg

FLAXSEED-CRUSTED CHICKEN TENDERS

Meal Description:

These Flaxseed-Crusted Chicken Tenders are a healthy and delicious alternative to traditional breaded chicken. The flaxseed coating adds a nutty flavor and a crunchy texture, making these chicken tenders a satisfying and nutritious choice for a family-friendly meal.

Ingredients:

For the Chicken Tenders:

- 1 lb chicken tenders
- 1/2 cup ground flaxseeds
- 1/4 cup grated Parmesan cheese
- One teaspoon of dried thyme
- One teaspoon of garlic powder
- 1/2 teaspoon onion powder
- Salt and black pepper to taste
- Cooking spray or olive oil for coating

For Dipping Sauce (Optional):

- 1/2 cup Greek yogurt
- One tablespoon of Dijon mustard
- One tablespoon honey
- One teaspoon of lemon juice
- Salt and black pepper to taste

Instructions:

1. Preheat the Oven:
   a. Preheat the oven to 400°F (200°C). Line a baking sheet with parchment paper or lightly grease it.
2. Prepare Coating Mixture:
   a. Combine ground flaxseeds, grated Parmesan cheese, dried thyme, garlic powder, onion powder, salt, and black pepper in a shallow bowl. Mix well to create the coating mixture.
3. Coat Chicken Tenders:
   a. Pat the chicken tenders dry with paper towels. Dip each chicken tender into the flaxseed mixture, ensuring an even coating on all sides. Press the mixture onto the chicken to adhere.
4. Place on Baking Sheet:
   a. Place the coated chicken tenders on the prepared baking sheet. Leave some space between each tender for even baking.
5. Spray or Brush with Oil:
   a. Lightly spray the tops of the chicken tenders with cooking spray or brush with olive oil. This helps achieve a

crispy crust.

6. Bake:

   a. Bake in the preheated oven for 20-25 minutes or until the chicken is cooked through and the coating is golden brown and crisp.

7. Prepare Dipping Sauce (Optional):

   a. Mix Greek yogurt, Dijon mustard, honey, lemon juice, salt, and black pepper in a small bowl to create a tangy dipping sauce.

8. Serve:

   a. Serve the Flaxseed-Crusted Chicken Tenders hot with the optional dipping sauce on the side.

9. Enjoy:

   a. Enjoy these nutritious and flavorful chicken tenders as a wholesome meal or a tasty snack.

Nutrition Information (Per Serving, without dipping sauce):

- Calories: 280
- Protein: 30g
- Fat: 15g
- Saturated Fat: 2.5g
- Carbohydrates: 5g
- Fiber: 4g
- Sugars: 0g
- Cholesterol: 75mg
- Sodium: 200mg

SALMON AND AVOCADO SUSHI ROLLS

Meal Description:

These Salmon and Avocado Sushi Rolls are a delicious and satisfying way to enjoy homemade sushi. The combination of fresh salmon, creamy avocado, and crisp cucumber wrapped in seasoned rice and nori creates a delightful balance of flavors and textures. Making sushi at home allows you to customize your rolls with your favorite ingredients.

Ingredients:

For the Sushi Rice:

• 2 cups sushi rice

• 2 1/2 cups water

• 1/2 cup rice vinegar

• Two tablespoons sugar

• One teaspoon salt

For the Sushi Rolls:

• Four sheets of nori (seaweed)

• 1/2 pound fresh salmon, thinly sliced

- One avocado, sliced
- One cucumber, julienned
- Soy sauce for dipping
- Pickled ginger and wasabi for serving (optional)

Instructions:

1. Prepare Sushi Rice:
   a. Rinse sushi rice under cold water until the water runs clear. In a rice cooker or on the stovetop, cook the rice with water according to package instructions.
   b. While the rice is still warm, gently fold in a mixture of rice vinegar, sugar, and salt. Allow the seasoned rice to cool to room temperature.
2. Assemble Sushi Rolls:
   a. Place a bamboo sushi rolling mat on a clean surface. Lay a sheet of nori, shiny side down, on the mat.
   b. Wet your hands to prevent the rice from sticking, and spread a thin layer of sushi rice over the nori, leaving a small border at the top.
3. Add Fillings:
   a. Arrange slices of fresh salmon, avocado, and julienned cucumber horizontally along the bottom edge of the nori.
4. Roll Sushi:
   a. Start rolling the sushi from the bottom using the bamboo mat, applying gentle pressure. Seal the edge with a bit of

water.

5. Slice Rolls:

   a. Slice the rolled sushi into bite-sized pieces with a sharp, wet knife.

6. Repeat:

   a. Repeat the process for the remaining nori sheets and fillings.

7. Serve:

   a. Arrange the Salmon and Avocado Sushi Rolls on a plate. Serve with soy sauce for dipping and, if desired, pickled ginger and wasabi on the side.

8. Enjoy:

   a. Enjoy your homemade sushi rolls as a delightful and customizable meal.

Note:

• You can add other ingredients like cream cheese, cucumber, or spicy mayo for additional flavor variations.

• Experiment with different sushi fillings to suit your taste preferences.

Nutrition Information (Per Serving, approximately six pieces):

• Calories: 350

• Protein: 15g

• Fat: 10g

• Saturated Fat: 2g

• Carbohydrates: 50g

• Fiber: 5g

• Sugars: 2g

- Cholesterol: 15mg
- Sodium: 600mg

ALMOND-CRUSTED TILAPIA WITH MANGO SALSA

Meal Description:

This Almond-Crusted Tilapia with Mango Salsa is a delightful and flavorful dish that combines the mild taste of tilapia with a crunchy almond crust and a vibrant mango salsa. It's a healthy and satisfying meal that's easy to prepare and perfect for a light dinner.

Ingredients:

For the Almond-Crusted Tilapia:

• Four tilapia fillets

• 1 cup almonds, finely chopped

• 1/2 cup whole wheat flour (or almond flour for a gluten-free option)

• Two eggs, beaten

• One teaspoon of smoked paprika

• Salt and black pepper to taste

• Olive oil for cooking

For the Mango Salsa:

- Two ripe mangoes, diced
- 1/2 red onion, finely chopped
- One red bell pepper, diced
- One jalapeño, seeds removed and finely chopped
- Juice of 1 lime
- 1/4 cup fresh cilantro, chopped
- Salt to taste

Instructions:

1. Preheat the Oven:
   a. Preheat the oven to 375°F (190°C).
2. Prepare Almond-Crusted Tilapia:
   a. Place the flour, beaten eggs, and chopped almonds mixed with smoked paprika, salt, and black pepper in three separate shallow dishes.
   b. Dredge each tilapia fillet in the flour, dip it into the beaten eggs, and coat it with the almond mixture, pressing the almonds onto the fillet to adhere.
3. Cook Tilapia:
   a. In an oven-safe skillet, heat olive oil over medium-high heat. Add the almond-crusted tilapia fillets and cook for 2-3 minutes on each side until golden brown.
   b. Transfer the skillet to the preheated oven and bake for an additional 10-12 minutes or until the tilapia is cooked through and flakes easily with a fork.
4. Prepare Mango Salsa:

      a. Combine diced mangoes, red onion, red bell pepper, jalapeño, lime juice, and chopped cilantro in a bowl. Mix well. Season with salt to taste.

5. Serve:

      a. Plate the almond-crusted tilapia and top each fillet with a generous scoop of mango salsa.

6. Enjoy:

      a. Enjoy this Almond-Crusted Tilapia with Mango Salsa as a delicious and nutritious dinner.

Nutrition Information (Per Serving):

- Calories: 400

- Protein: 30g

- Fat: 22g

- Saturated Fat: 2g

- Carbohydrates: 25g

- Fiber: 6g

- Sugars: 12g

- Cholesterol: 80mg

- Sodium: 120mg

SESAME GINGER SALMON SKEWERS

Meal Description:

These Sesame Ginger Salmon Skewers are a mouthwatering and flavorful dish that combines the rich taste of salmon with the zing of ginger and the nuttiness of sesame. Grilled to perfection, these skewers make for a delightful and healthy meal with a perfect balance of savory and tangy flavors.

Ingredients:

For the Salmon Skewers:

• 1 lb salmon fillets, skinless, cut into cubes

• Two tablespoons soy sauce (low sodium)

• One tablespoon of sesame oil

• One tablespoon of rice vinegar

• One tablespoon honey

• One tablespoon of fresh ginger, grated

• Two cloves garlic, minced

• One tablespoon of sesame seeds (for garnish)

• Wooden skewers soaked in water for at least 30 minutes

For Serving:

- Cooked brown rice or quinoa
- Sliced green onions (for garnish)
- Lime wedges

Instructions:

1. Prepare Marinade:
   a. In a bowl, whisk together soy sauce, sesame oil, rice vinegar, honey, grated ginger, and minced garlic to create the marinade.
2. Marinate Salmon:
   a. Cut the salmon fillets into cubes. Place the salmon cubes in a shallow dish and pour the marinade over them. Ensure the salmon is well-coated. Cover and refrigerate for at least 30 minutes to let the flavors infuse.
3. Thread Salmon onto Skewers:
   a. Preheat the grill. Thread the marinated salmon cubes onto the soaked wooden skewers.
4. Grill Salmon Skewers:
   a. Grill the salmon skewers over medium-high heat for about 3-4 minutes per side or until the salmon is cooked through and has an excellent grill mark.
5. Garnish:
   a. Remove the skewers from the grill and place them on a serving platter. Sprinkle sesame seeds over the top for garnish.
6. Serve:
   a. Serve the Sesame Ginger Salmon Skewers over cooked brown rice or

quinoa. Garnish with sliced green onions and serve with lime wedges on the side.

7. Enjoy:

    a. Enjoy this delightful and flavorful dish that brings together the goodness of salmon and the exotic taste of sesame and ginger.

Nutrition Information (Per Serving, excluding rice/quinoa):

- Calories: 280

- Protein: 25g

- Fat: 15g

- Saturated Fat: 2.5g

- Carbohydrates: 10g

- Fiber: 1g

- Sugars: 7g

- Cholesterol: 60mg

- Sodium: 400mg

MACKEREL AND QUINOA SALAD

Meal Description:

This Mackerel and Quinoa Salad is a nutrient-packed dish that combines the robust flavors of mackerel with the wholesome goodness of quinoa and a medley of fresh vegetables. It's a satisfying and protein-rich salad that makes for a delicious and nutritious meal.

Ingredients:

For the Salad:

- 1 cup quinoa, cooked and cooled
- Two cans (about 8 oz each) of mackerel fillets in olive oil, drained
- 1 cup cherry tomatoes, halved
- One cucumber, diced
- 1/2 red onion, finely chopped
- 1/4 cup Kalamata olives, pitted and sliced
- 1/4 cup fresh parsley, chopped

For the Dressing:

- Three tablespoons extra-virgin olive oil
- Two tablespoons of red wine vinegar

- One teaspoon of Dijon mustard
- One clove of garlic, minced
- Salt and black pepper to taste

Instructions:

1. Prepare Quinoa:
   a. Cook quinoa according to package instructions. Once cooked, fluff it with a fork and let it cool to room temperature.
2. Prepare Dressing:
   a. Whisk together extra-virgin olive oil, red wine vinegar, Dijon mustard, minced garlic, salt, and black pepper in a small bowl. Set aside.
3. Assemble Salad:
   a. In a large mixing bowl, combine the cooked and cooled quinoa with mackerel fillets (broken into chunks), cherry tomatoes, diced cucumber, chopped red onion, sliced Kalamata olives, and fresh parsley.
4. Add Dressing:
   a. Pour the prepared dressing over the salad ingredients. Gently toss the salad until all ingredients are well-coated with the dressing.
5. Chill (Optional):
   a. For enhanced flavors, refrigerate the salad for 30 minutes before serving.
6. Serve:
   a. Serve the Mackerel and Quinoa Salad in individual bowls or on a platter.
7. Enjoy:

a. Enjoy this flavorful and protein-packed salad as a wholesome and satisfying meal.

Note:

• You can customize the salad by adding other vegetables like bell peppers or avocado.

• Adjust the dressing ingredients to suit your taste preferences.

Nutrition Information (Per Serving):

• Calories: 400

• Protein: 25g

• Fat: 20g

• Saturated Fat: 3g

• Carbohydrates: 30g

• Fiber: 5g

• Sugars: 2g

• Cholesterol: 30mg

• Sodium: 400mg

TUNA AND WHITE BEAN SALAD

Meal Description:

This Tuna and White Bean Salad is a refreshing and protein-packed dish that combines the goodness of tuna, white beans, and a variety of fresh vegetables. The zesty lemon vinaigrette combines all the flavors, making it a light and satisfying salad perfect for a quick and nutritious meal.

Ingredients:

For the Salad:

• Two cans (about 5 oz each) of tuna in water, drained

• Two cans (about 15 oz each) of cannellini beans, drained and rinsed

• 1 cup cherry tomatoes, halved

• 1/2 red onion, finely chopped

• One cucumber, diced

• 1/4 cup Kalamata olives, pitted and sliced

• 1/4 cup fresh parsley, chopped

• 1/4 cup feta cheese, crumbled (optional)

For the Lemon Vinaigrette:

- Three tablespoons extra-virgin olive oil
- Juice of 1 lemon
- One teaspoon of Dijon mustard
- One clove of garlic, minced
- Salt and black pepper to taste

Instructions:

1. Prepare Tuna and Beans:
   a. In a large mixing bowl, combine drained tuna and rinsed cannellini beans.
2. Add Vegetables:
   a. Add cherry tomatoes, chopped red onion, diced cucumber, sliced Kalamata olives, and chopped fresh parsley to the bowl.
3. Prepare Lemon Vinaigrette:
   a. Whisk together extra-virgin olive oil, lemon juice, Dijon mustard, minced garlic, salt, and black pepper in a small bowl to create the lemon vinaigrette.
4. Pour Dressing:
   a. Pour the lemon vinaigrette over the tuna and vegetable mixture.
5. Toss Gently:
   a. Gently toss the salad to ensure that all ingredients are well-coated with the dressing.
6. Chill (Optional):
   a. For enhanced flavors, refrigerate the salad for 30 minutes before serving.
7. Top with Feta (Optional):
   a. If desired, sprinkle crumbled feta cheese

over the top before serving.

8. Serve:
    a. Serve the Tuna and White Bean Salad in individual bowls or on a platter.

9. Enjoy:
    a. Enjoy this light and protein-packed salad as a nutritious and satisfying meal.

Note:

• You can customize the salad by adding other vegetables like bell peppers, cherry tomatoes, or avocado.

• Adjust the dressing ingredients to suit your taste preferences.

Nutrition Information (Per Serving):

• Calories: 350

• Protein: 25g

• Fat: 15g

• Saturated Fat: 2.5g

• Carbohydrates: 30g

• Fiber: 8g

• Sugars: 2g

• Cholesterol: 30mg

• Sodium: 600mg

BAKED TROUT WITH LEMON AND HERBS

Meal Description:

This Baked Trout with Lemon and Herbs is a simple and elegant dish highlighting trout's delicate flavor. The combination of zesty lemon, aromatic herbs, and tender fish creates a delightful and healthy meal that's easy to prepare.

Ingredients:

For the Baked Trout:

- Four trout fillets (about 6 oz each), scaled and cleaned
- Two tablespoons of olive oil
- Two lemons, thinly sliced
- Three cloves garlic, minced
- Two tablespoons fresh parsley, chopped
- One tablespoon of fresh dill, chopped
- Salt and black pepper to taste

Instructions:

1. Preheat the Oven:

    a. Preheat the oven to 400°F (200°C).

2. Prepare Trout Fillets:
   a. Pat the trout fillets dry with paper towels. Place them on a baking sheet lined with parchment paper.
3. Season Trout:
   a. Drizzle olive oil over the trout fillets, ensuring they are well-coated. Season with salt and black pepper to taste.
4. Add Lemon and Herbs:
   a. Place thin lemon slices on top of each trout fillet. Sprinkle minced garlic, chopped fresh parsley, and chopped fresh dill over the fish.
5. Bake:
   a. Bake in the preheated oven for 15-20 minutes or until the trout is cooked through and flakes easily with a fork.
6. Broil (Optional):
   a. If you desire a slightly crispy top, you can switch to the broil setting for the last 2-3 minutes of cooking.
7. Serve:
   a. Carefully transfer the Baked Trout with Lemon and Herbs to serving plates.
8. Garnish (Optional):
   a. Garnish with additional fresh herbs and lemon wedges for a burst of citrus flavor.
9. Enjoy:
   a. Enjoy this light and flavorful Baked Trout as a delicious and nutritious main course.

10. Note:
   a. You can customize the herb selection based on your preferences. Thyme or rosemary also work well with trout.
   b. Pair the baked trout with a side of roasted vegetables or a light salad for a well-balanced meal.

Nutrition Information (Per Serving):

- Calories: 250

- Protein: 30g

- Fat: 12g

- Saturated Fat: 2g

- Carbohydrates: 6g

- Fiber: 2g

- Sugars: 1g

- Cholesterol: 60mg

- Sodium: 80mg

OMEGA-3 SMOOTHIE WITH KALE AND PINEAPPLE

Smoothie Description:

This Omega-3 Smoothie with Kale and Pineapple is a delicious and nutritious way to boost your omega-3 fatty acids, vitamins, and antioxidants intake. Combining kale, pineapple, chia seeds, and flaxseed oil creates a vibrant and refreshing smoothie and provides essential nutrients for overall well-being.

Ingredients:

- 1 cup kale leaves, stems removed
- 1 cup fresh pineapple chunks
- One banana, peeled
- One tablespoon of chia seeds
- One tablespoon of flaxseed oil
- 1/2 cup Greek yogurt (optional for creaminess)
- 1 cup coconut water or almond milk
- Ice cubes (optional)

Instructions:

1. Prepare Ingredients:
   a. Wash the kale leaves thoroughly, remove the stems, and roughly chop them.
   b. Peel and chop the fresh pineapple into chunks.
   c. Peel the banana.
2. Assemble in Blender:
   a. In a blender, combine the chopped kale, pineapple chunks, banana, chia seeds, flaxseed oil, and Greek yogurt (if using).
3. Add Liquid:
   a. Pour in the coconut water or almond milk.
4. Blend Until Smooth:
   a. Blend all the ingredients until smooth and creamy. If the smoothie is too thick, you can add more liquid to achieve your desired consistency.
5. Check Consistency:
   a. Add ice cubes if you prefer a colder and thicker smoothie. Blend again until the ice is well incorporated.
6. Serve:
   a. Pour the Omega-3 Smoothie with Kale and Pineapple into a glass.
7. Garnish (Optional):
   a. Garnish with a pineapple wedge or a sprinkle of chia seeds for an extra touch.
8. Enjoy:
   a. Sip and enjoy this refreshing and nutrient-packed smoothie, rich in

omega-3 fatty acids and essential vitamins.

Note:

• Add more or less fruit, yogurt, or liquid to adjust the sweetness and thickness.

• You can use frozen pineapple chunks for a colder smoothie.

Nutrition Information (Approximate Values):

• Calories: 250

• Protein: 7g

• Fat: 10g

• Saturated Fat: 1g

• Carbohydrates: 35g

• Fiber: 7g

• Sugars: 18g

• Omega-3 Fatty Acids: 2.5g

CHAPTER FIVE

Antioxidant-Rich Foods Recipes
Berry and Spinach Smoothie Bowl

Smoothie Bowl Description:

This Berry and Spinach Smoothie Bowl is visually appealing and packed with antioxidants, vitamins, and minerals. The combination of mixed berries, spinach, and wholesome toppings creates a delicious and nutritious breakfast or snack that's as enjoyable to eat as it is beneficial for your health.

Ingredients:

For the Smoothie Base:

• 1 cup mixed berries (strawberries, blueberries, raspberries)

• One banana, frozen

• 1 cup fresh spinach leaves

• 1/2 cup Greek yogurt

• 1/2 cup almond milk

• One tablespoon of chia seeds (optional for thickness)

• One tablespoon of honey or maple syrup (optional for sweetness)

• Ice cubes (optional)

Toppings:

• Sliced strawberries

• Blueberries

• Granola

• Chia seeds

- Shredded coconut
- Drizzle of honey

Instructions:

1. Prepare Ingredients:
   a. If not using frozen berries, ensure the banana is frozen for a creamier texture.
2. Blend Smoothie Base:
   a. Combine mixed berries, frozen banana, fresh spinach, Greek yogurt, almond milk, chia seeds (if using), and honey or maple syrup (if desired). Blend until smooth and creamy.
3. Check Consistency:
   a. Add ice cubes if you prefer a thicker consistency. Blend again until the ice is well incorporated.
4. Pour into Bowl:
   a. Pour the smoothie into a bowl, ensuring a smooth and even surface.
5. Add Toppings:
   a. Arrange sliced strawberries, blueberries, granola, chia seeds, and shredded coconut on top of the smoothie bowl.
6. Drizzle Honey (Optional):
   a. For added sweetness, drizzle honey over the toppings.
7. Serve Immediately:
   a. Serve the Berry and Spinach Smoothie Bowl immediately and enjoy the burst of flavors and textures.

Note:

• Customize your toppings based on personal preferences. Add nuts, seeds, or other fruits for variety.

• Adjust the sweetness by adding more or less honey or maple syrup.

Nutrition Information (Approximate Values):

• Calories: 350

• Protein: 12g

• Fat: 8g

• Saturated Fat: 2g

• Carbohydrates: 60g

• Fiber: 10g

• Sugars: 35g

BLUEBERRY AND WALNUT OATMEAL

Oatmeal Description:

This Blueberry and Walnut Oatmeal is a wholesome and nutritious breakfast option that combines the goodness of whole grains, fresh blueberries, and crunchy walnuts. Packed with fiber, antioxidants, and omega-3 fatty acids, this oatmeal is delicious and a great way to start your day on a healthy note.

Ingredients:

• 1/2 cup old-fashioned rolled oats

• 1 cup milk (dairy or plant-based)

• 1/2 cup fresh blueberries

• Two tablespoons chopped walnuts

• One tablespoon of honey or maple syrup (optional for sweetness)

• 1/2 teaspoon vanilla extract

• Pinch of salt

Instructions:

1. Cook Oats:
    a. In a saucepan, combine old-fashioned rolled oats and milk. Bring to a gentle

boil over medium heat.
2. Simmer:
   a. Reduce the heat to low and simmer, stirring occasionally, until the oats are tender and the mixture has thickened (about 5-7 minutes).
3. Add Blueberries:
   a. Add fresh blueberries to the cooking oats. Stir well to incorporate them into the oatmeal.
4. Flavor with Vanilla:
   a. Stir in vanilla extract and a pinch of salt for added flavor. Adjust sweetness by adding honey or maple syrup if desired.
5. Serve:
   a. Once the oatmeal reaches your preferred consistency, remove it from heat.
6. Top with Walnuts:
   a. Sprinkle chopped walnuts over the top of the oatmeal for a delightful crunch.
7. Drizzle Sweetener (Optional):
   a. If desired, drizzle honey or maple syrup over the Blueberry and Walnut Oatmeal for added sweetness.
8. Enjoy Warm:
   a. Serve the oatmeal warm in a bowl, and enjoy a nutritious and satisfying breakfast.

Note:

• Feel free to customize the toppings with additional fruits, seeds, or a dollop of yogurt.

· Adjust the thickness of the oatmeal by adding more or less milk based on your preference.

Nutrition Information (Approximate Values):

· Calories: 350

· Protein: 10g

· Fat: 15g

· Saturated Fat: 2g

· Carbohydrates: 45g

· Fiber: 7g

· Sugars: 15g

KALE AND BERRY SALAD WITH GOAT CHEESE

Salad Description:

This Kale and Berry Salad with Goat Cheese is a vibrant and nutritious dish that combines kale's earthy flavor with the sweetness of mixed berries and the creamy tang of goat cheese. Tossed in a light balsamic vinaigrette, this salad perfectly balances flavors and textures, making it a delightful addition to any meal.

Ingredients:

For the Salad:

• 4 cups kale leaves, stems removed and thinly sliced

• 1 cup mixed berries (strawberries, blueberries, raspberries)

• 1/2 cup crumbled goat cheese

• 1/4 cup sliced almonds, toasted

For the Balsamic Vinaigrette:

• Three tablespoons extra-virgin olive oil

• Two tablespoons of balsamic vinegar

• One teaspoon of Dijon mustard

- One clove of garlic, minced
- Salt and black pepper to taste

Instructions:

1. Prepare Kale:
   a. Wash the kale leaves thoroughly, remove the stems, and thinly slice them.
2. Toast Almonds:
   a. In a dry skillet over medium heat, toast the sliced almonds until they are golden brown. Stir frequently to prevent burning. Remove from heat and let them cool.
3. Prepare Vinaigrette:
   a. Whisk together extra-virgin olive oil, balsamic vinegar, Dijon mustard, minced garlic, salt, and black pepper in a small bowl to create the balsamic Vinaigrette.
4. Massage Kale:
   a. Place the sliced kale in a large bowl. Pour half of the balsamic Vinaigrette over the kale. Using your hands, massage the kale for a few minutes until it becomes tender.
5. Assemble Salad:
   a. Add the mixed berries, crumbled goat cheese, and toasted sliced almonds to the kale.
6. Drizzle remaining Vinaigrette:
   a. Drizzle the remaining balsamic Vinaigrette over the salad.
7. Toss Gently:

a. Toss the salad gently to ensure all ingredients are well-coated with the Vinaigrette.

8. Serve:

a. Serve the Kale and Berry Salad with Goat Cheese on individual plates or in a large salad bowl.

9. Enjoy:

a. Enjoy this refreshing and nutrient-packed salad as a side or a light main course.

Note:

• Customize the salad by adding other fruits, such as sliced peaches or pomegranate seeds.

• Adjust the vinaigrette ingredients to suit your taste preferences.

Nutrition Information (Approximate Values):

• Calories: 300

• Protein: 10g

• Fat: 20g

• Saturated Fat: 6g

• Carbohydrates: 25g

• Fiber: 6g

• Sugars: 10g

• Cholesterol: 15mg

• Sodium: 200mg

ROASTED VEGETABLE MEDLEY WITH HERBS

Dish Description:

This Roasted Vegetable Medley with Herbs is a colorful and flavorful side dish that brings out the natural sweetness and savory goodness of a variety of vegetables. Roasted to perfection with a blend of herbs, this medley makes a delicious and nutritious addition to any meal.

Ingredients:

For the Roasted Vegetables:

• 2 cups cherry tomatoes, halved

• One bell pepper (red or yellow), diced

• One zucchini, sliced into rounds

• One yellow squash, sliced into rounds

• One red onion, cut into wedges

• 1 cup baby carrots, halved lengthwise

• Two tablespoons of olive oil

- One teaspoon of dried thyme
- One teaspoon of dried rosemary
- One teaspoon dried oregano
- Salt and black pepper to taste

Instructions:

1. Preheat Oven:
   a. Preheat the oven to 400°F (200°C).
2. Prepare Vegetables:
   a. Combine halved cherry tomatoes, diced bell pepper, sliced zucchini, yellow squash, onion wedges, and halved baby carrots in a large mixing bowl.
3. Coat with Olive Oil:
   a. Drizzle olive oil over the vegetables. Toss the vegetables to ensure they are evenly coated with the oil.
4. Season with Herbs:
   a. Sprinkle dried thyme, rosemary, oregano, salt, and black pepper over the vegetables. Toss again to distribute the herbs evenly.
5. Arrange on Baking Sheet:
   a. Spread the seasoned vegetables in a single layer on a baking sheet. Ensure they are not overcrowded to allow for even roasting.
6. Roast in Oven:
   a. Roast the vegetables in the preheated oven for 25-30 minutes or until they are tender and golden brown, stirring halfway through the cooking time.

7. Check for Doneness:
   a. Check the doneness of the vegetables by inserting a fork or knife into a few pieces. They should be fork-tenders.
8. Serve:
   a. Transfer the Roasted Vegetable Medley with Herbs to a serving platter.
9. Garnish (Optional):
   a. Garnish with fresh herbs, such as chopped parsley or basil, if desired.
10. Enjoy:
   a. Serve this flavorful and vibrant vegetable medley as a side dish to complement your main course.

Note:

• You can customize the selection of vegetables based on your preferences or what's in season.

• Experiment with different herb combinations to suit your taste.

Nutrition Information (Approximate Values):

• Calories: 150

• Protein: 3g

• Fat: 8g

• Saturated Fat: 1g

• Carbohydrates: 20g

• Fiber: 5g

• Sugars: 8g

• Sodium: 50mg

DARK CHOCOLATE AND MIXED BERRY PARFAIT

Parfait Description:

This Dark Chocolate and Mixed Berry Parfait is a decadent yet wholesome dessert that combines the richness of dark chocolate with the freshness of mixed berries. Layered with creamy Greek yogurt and crunchy granola, it's a delightful treat that satisfies both your sweet cravings and your desire for a balanced indulgence.

Ingredients:

• 1 cup mixed berries (strawberries, blueberries, raspberries)

• 1 cup Greek yogurt (vanilla or plain)

• 1/2 cup dark chocolate chips or chunks

• 1/2 cup granola (homemade or store-bought)

• Two tablespoons honey or maple syrup (optional for drizzling)

• Fresh mint leaves for garnish (optional)

Instructions:

    1. Prepare Berries:

    a. Wash and prepare the mixed berries. If using strawberries, hull and slice them.

2. Melt Dark Chocolate:

    a. In a microwave-safe bowl or using a double boiler, melt the dark chocolate chips or chunks until smooth. Stir frequently to prevent burning.

3. Layering:

    a. In serving glasses or bowls, start by adding a layer of Greek yogurt at the bottom.

4. Add Berries:

    a. Add a layer of mixed berries on top of the yogurt.

5. Drizzle Chocolate:

    a. Drizzle a portion of the melted dark chocolate over the berries.

6. Sprinkle Granola:

    a. Sprinkle a layer of granola over the chocolate.

7. Repeat Layers:

    a. Repeat the layering process until you reach the top of the glass, finishing with a final drizzle of dark chocolate.

8. Garnish (Optional):

    a. Garnish the Dark Chocolate and Mixed Berry Parfait with fresh mint leaves for a burst of freshness.

9. Serve Chilled:

    a. Place the parfaits in the refrigerator for at least 30 minutes to allow the layers to set and the flavors to meld.

10. Drizzle Honey (Optional):

a. Drizzle honey or maple syrup over the top just before serving for added sweetness if desired.

11. Enjoy:

a. Enjoy this luscious Dark Chocolate and Mixed Berry Parfait as a delightful and satisfying dessert.

Note:

• Customize the parfait by adding other fruits or incorporating different types of chocolate.

• Adjust the sweetness by using flavored yogurt or varying the amount of honey or maple syrup.

Nutrition Information (Approximate Values):

• Calories: 350

• Protein: 15g

• Fat: 15g

• Saturated Fat: 8g

• Carbohydrates: 45g

• Fiber: 7g

• Sugars: 25g

BROCCOLI AND CAULIFLOWER SALAD WITH CRANBERRIES

Salad Description:

This Broccoli and Cauliflower Salad with Cranberries is a refreshing and crunchy dish that balances the nutty flavors of broccoli and cauliflower with the sweetness of dried cranberries. Tossed in a light and tangy dressing, this salad is delicious and a vibrant addition to any meal.

Ingredients:

For the Salad:

• 2 cups broccoli florets, blanched

• 2 cups cauliflower florets, blanched

• 1/2 cup dried cranberries

• 1/4 cup red onion, finely chopped

• 1/4 cup sunflower seeds or slivered almonds, toasted

For the Dressing:

• 1/3 cup mayonnaise

- Two tablespoons Greek yogurt (optional for creaminess)
- Two tablespoons of apple cider vinegar
- One tablespoon of honey or maple syrup
- Salt and black pepper to taste

Instructions:

1. Blanch Broccoli and Cauliflower:
    a. Bring a pot of water to boil. Add broccoli and cauliflower florets and blanch for 2 minutes. Drain and immediately transfer the florets to ice water to stop the cooking process. Drain again and pat them dry.
2. Prepare Salad Base:
    a. Combine blanched broccoli and cauliflower florets, dried cranberries, chopped red onion, and toasted sunflower seeds or slivered almonds in a large bowl.
3. Prepare Dressing:
    a. In a small bowl, whisk together mayonnaise, Greek yogurt (if using), apple cider vinegar, honey or maple syrup, salt, and black pepper to create the dressing.
4. Toss Salad:
    a. Pour the dressing over the salad ingredients. Toss gently to ensure all components are well-coated with the dressing.
5. Chill (Optional):
    a. Refrigerate the Broccoli and Cauliflower

Salad for at least 30 minutes before serving to allow the flavors to meld.

6. Serve:
   a. Serve the chilled salad in individual bowls or on a platter.
7. Enjoy:
   a. Enjoy this vibrant and nutritious Broccoli and Cauliflower Salad with Cranberries as a side dish or a light meal.

Note:

• Add ingredients like shredded cheese, bacon bits, or cherry tomatoes to customize the salad.

• Adjust the sweetness and tanginess of the dressing according to your taste preferences.

Nutrition Information (Approximate Values):

• Calories: 250

• Protein: 5g

• Fat: 18g

• Saturated Fat: 3g

• Carbohydrates: 20g

• Fiber: 5g

• Sugars: 10g

• Sodium: 150mg

GREEN TEA INFUSED QUINOA

Quinoa Description:

This Green Tea Infused Quinoa is a unique and flavorful twist on traditional quinoa, combining the nuttiness of quinoa with the subtle earthy notes of green tea. This versatile and nutritious dish can be enjoyed as a side or base for various meals, adding a touch of sophistication to your plate.

Ingredients:

• 1 cup quinoa, rinsed

• 2 cups water

• One green tea bag (sencha or your preferred green tea variety)

• 1/2 teaspoon salt

• Optional: Chopped fresh herbs (such as parsley or cilantro) for garnish

Instructions:

1. Brew Green Tea:
   a. In a saucepan, bring 2 cups of water to a boil. Add the green tea bag to the boiling water and let it steep for 3-5 minutes. Remove the tea bag and discard.

2. Add Quinoa:
   a. Rinse the quinoa under cold water. Add the rinsed quinoa to the brewed green tea.
3. Cook Quinoa:
   a. Bring the green tea and quinoa mixture to a boil. Reduce the heat to low, cover the saucepan, and simmer for 15-20 minutes or until the quinoa is cooked and the liquid is absorbed.
4. Fluff Quinoa:
   a. Once cooked, fluff the quinoa with a fork to separate the grains.
5. Season with Salt:
   a. Stir in the salt to taste. Adjust the seasoning if needed.
6. Garnish (Optional):
   a. Garnish the Green Tea Infused Quinoa with chopped fresh herbs, such as parsley or cilantro, for added freshness.
7. Serve Warm:
   a. Serve the quinoa warm as a delightful and aromatic side dish.

Note:

• Experiment with different green tea varieties to explore varied flavor profiles.

• Use the Green Tea Infused Quinoa as a base for salads and Buddha bowls or as a side for grilled proteins.

Nutrition Information (Approximate Values):

• Calories: 200

• Protein: 8g

- Fat: 3g
- Saturated Fat: 0g
- Carbohydrates: 38g
- Fiber: 4g
- Sugars: 0g
- Sodium: 300mg

POMEGRANATE AND PISTACHIO QUINOA SALAD

Salad Description:

This Pomegranate and Pistachio Quinoa Salad is a vibrant and nutritious dish that combines the nuttiness of quinoa with the sweet and tart flavors of pomegranate seeds and the crunch of pistachios. Tossed in a citrusy vinaigrette, this salad is visually appealing and a delightful addition to any meal.

Ingredients:

For the Salad:

- 1 cup quinoa, rinsed

- 2 cups water

- 1 cup pomegranate seeds

- 1/2 cup shelled pistachios, chopped

- 1/4 cup red onion, finely chopped

- 1/4 cup fresh parsley, chopped

For the Citrus Vinaigrette:

- Three tablespoons extra-virgin olive oil

- Juice of 1 lemon
- Juice of 1 orange
- One teaspoon of Dijon mustard
- One teaspoon of honey or maple syrup
- Salt and black pepper to taste

Instructions:

1. Cook Quinoa:
   a. In a saucepan, combine the rinsed quinoa and water. Bring to a boil, then reduce heat to low, cover, and simmer for 15-20 minutes or until the quinoa is cooked and the water is absorbed. Fluff with a fork and let it cool.
2. Prepare Vinaigrette:
   a. Whisk together extra-virgin olive oil, lemon juice, orange juice, Dijon mustard, honey or maple syrup, salt, and black pepper in a small bowl to create the citrus vinaigrette.
3. Assemble Salad:
   a. Combine the cooked quinoa, pomegranate seeds, chopped pistachios, finely chopped red onion, and chopped fresh parsley in a large bowl.
4. Pour Vinaigrette:
   a. Pour the citrus vinaigrette over the salad.
5. Toss Gently:
   a. Gently toss the salad to ensure all ingredients are well-coated with the Vinaigrette.

6. Chill (Optional):
   a. Refrigerate the Pomegranate and Pistachio Quinoa Salad for 30 minutes before serving to enhance the flavors.
7. Serve:
   a. Serve the salad in individual bowls or on a platter.
8. Enjoy:
   a. Enjoy this colorful and flavorful quinoa salad as a refreshing side or a light and wholesome main dish.

Note:

• Customize the salad by adding crumbled feta or goat cheese for added creaminess.

• Adjust the sweetness and acidity of the Vinaigrette according to your taste.

Nutrition Information (Approximate Values):

• Calories: 300

• Protein: 8g

• Fat: 15g

• Saturated Fat: 2g

• Carbohydrates: 35g

• Fiber: 6g

• Sugars: 6g

• Sodium: 150mg

RASPBERRY AND ALMOND BUTTER TOAST

Toast Description:

This Raspberry and Almond Butter Toast is a simple yet delightful combination of creamy almond butter, fresh raspberries, and a drizzle of honey on toasted whole-grain bread. This toast perfectly balances nutty, fruity, and sweet flavors, making it a satisfying and wholesome breakfast or snack.

Ingredients:

- Two slices of whole-grain bread toasted
- Four tablespoons of almond butter
- 1 cup fresh raspberries
- Honey for drizzling
- Optional: Sliced almonds for garnish

Instructions:

1. Toast-Bread:
   a. Toast the whole-grain bread slices to your desired level of crispiness.
2. Spread Almond Butter:

       a. Spread a generous layer of almond butter evenly on each toasted bread slice.

3. Add Raspberries:

       a. Arrange fresh raspberries on top of the almond butter layer. Press them slightly to adhere to the almond butter.

4. Drizzle Honey:

       a. Drizzle honey over the raspberries for added sweetness. Use as much or as little honey as desired.

5. Optional Garnish:

       a. Garnish the Raspberry and Almond Butter Toast with sliced almonds for an extra crunch.

6. Serve:

       a. Serve the toast immediately while it's still warm.

7. Enjoy:

       a. Enjoy this delightful and nutritious Raspberry and Almond Butter Toast as a quick and satisfying breakfast or snack.

Note:

• For variety, experiment with different types of nut butter, such as peanut butter or cashew butter.

• Consider adding a sprinkle of chia seeds or flaxseeds for an additional nutritional boost.

Nutrition Information (Approximate Values):

• Calories: 350

• Protein: 10g

• Fat: 20g

- Saturated Fat: 2g
- Carbohydrates: 40g
- Fiber: 8g
- Sugars: 12g
- Sodium: 200mg

MIXED BERRIES AND GREEK YOGURT POPSICLES

Popsicle Description:

These Mixed Berries and Greek Yogurt Popsicles are a refreshing and wholesome treat, combining the natural sweetness of mixed berries with the creamy goodness of Greek yogurt. These homemade popsicles are not only delicious but also a nutritious option for an excellent and satisfying dessert or snack.

Ingredients:

• 1 cup mixed berries (strawberries, blueberries, raspberries)

• 1 cup Greek yogurt (vanilla or plain)

• Two tablespoons of honey or maple syrup

• One teaspoon of vanilla extract

Instructions:

    1. Prepare Berries:

        a. Wash and hull strawberries if using.

Combine the mixed berries in a bowl.
2. Blend Berries:
   a. In a blender, puree the mixed berries until smooth. If desired, strain the puree to remove seeds for a smoother texture.
3. Sweeten and Flavor Yogurt:
   a. Mix Greek yogurt with honey or maple syrup and vanilla extract in a separate bowl. Adjust sweetness to taste.
4. Layer in Popsicle Molds:
   a. Spoon a layer of the berry puree into popsicle molds, filling each mold about one-third full.
5. Add Yogurt Layer:
   a. Add a layer of sweetened Greek yogurt on top of the berry puree, filling the molds to about two-thirds full.
6. Top with More Berries:
   a. Spoon additional berry puree on top of the yogurt layer, filling the molds to the top.
7. Swirl with a Stick:
   a. Insert a popsicle stick into each mold and gently swirl it to create a marbled effect.
8. Freeze:
   a. Place the popsicle molds in the freezer and freeze for at least 4-6 hours or until the popsicles are completely set.
9. Unmold Popsicles:
   a. Once fully frozen, remove the popsicle molds from the freezer. To unmold, briefly run the molds under warm water

to release the popsicles.

10. Serve and Enjoy:

    a. Serve these Mixed Berries and Greek Yogurt Popsicles for a delightful and nutritious frozen treat.

Note:

• Customize the popsicles with your favorite berries, or use a single-berry variety for simplicity.

• Experiment with different flavors of Greek yogurt, such as honey or fruit-flavored varieties.

Nutrition Information (Approximate Values):

• Calories: 80

• Protein: 4g

• Fat: 2g

• Saturated Fat: 1g

• Carbohydrates: 12g

• Fiber: 2g

• Sugars: 8g

• Sodium: 20mg

CHAPTER SIX

Hydration Recipes
Hydrating Green Smoothie with Cucumber and Kale

Smoothie Description:

This Hydrating Green Smoothie with Cucumber and Kale is a refreshing and nutrient-packed beverage that combines cucumber's hydrating properties with kale's nutritional benefits. Packed with vitamins, minerals, and antioxidants, this green smoothie is delicious and an excellent choice for a hydrating and revitalizing drink.

Ingredients:

- 1 cup cucumber, peeled and sliced
- 1 cup kale leaves, stems removed
- 1/2 green apple, cored and chopped
- 1/2 banana, peeled
- 1/2 lemon, juiced
- 1 cup coconut water (or plain water)
- One tablespoon of chia seeds
- Ice cubes (optional)

Instructions:

1. Prepare Ingredients:
    a. Peel and slice the cucumber. Remove the stems from the kale leaves. Core and chop the green apple. Peel the banana.
2. Juice Lemon:
    a. Juice half a lemon to add a citrusy zing to the smoothie.
3. Blend Smoothie:

     a. Combine cucumber, kale leaves, green apple, banana, lemon juice, and chia seeds in a blender.

4. Add Coconut Water:

     a. Pour coconut water (or plain water) into the blender.

5. Blend Until Smooth:

     a. Blend the ingredients until smooth and creamy. Add ice cubes and blend again for a colder and icier consistency if desired.

6. Check Consistency:

     a. Adjust the thickness of the smoothie by adding more water if needed. Blend until the desired consistency is achieved.

7. Pour and Serve:

     a. Pour the Hydrating Green Smoothie into a glass.

8. Garnish (Optional):

     a. Garnish with a slice of cucumber or a sprinkle of chia seeds if desired.

9. Enjoy:

     a. Enjoy this Hydrating Green Smoothie as a revitalizing and hydrating drink, perfect for any time of the day.

Note:

• Customize the smoothie by adding a handful of mint leaves for extra freshness.

• You can include a tablespoon of honey or maple syrup for added sweetness.

Nutrition Information (Approximate Values):

- Calories: 150
- Protein: 4g
- Fat: 3g
- Saturated Fat: 1g
- Carbohydrates: 30g
- Fiber: 8g
- Sugars: 15g
- Sodium: 50mg

ICED GINGER MINT GREEN TEA

Tea Description:

This Iced Ginger Mint Green Tea is a refreshing and invigorating beverage that combines the earthy notes of green tea with the zesty kick of ginger and the cool freshness of mint. Perfect for warm days or as a pick-me-up, this iced tea is a delightful way to enjoy the health benefits of green tea with a twist of flavor.

Ingredients:

• Two green tea bags

• 1-inch piece of fresh ginger, thinly sliced

• Handful of fresh mint leaves

• 1-2 tablespoons honey or maple syrup (optional for sweetness)

• Ice cubes

• Lemon slices for garnish (optional)

Instructions:

1. Brew Green Tea:
   a. Place the green tea bags in a heatproof pitcher. Boil water and pour it over the tea bags. Allow the tea to steep for 3-5

minutes.
2. Add Ginger Slices:
   a. Add thinly sliced ginger to the hot tea. This adds a zesty and warming flavor.
3. Cool Tea:
   a. Let the tea cool to room temperature. You can speed up the process by placing it in the refrigerator for a faster chill.
4. Add Mint Leaves:
   a. Once the tea has cooled, add a handful of fresh mint leaves. This will infuse the tea with a refreshing, minty flavor.
5. Sweeten (Optional):
   a. If desired, add honey or maple syrup to sweeten the tea. Adjust the sweetness to your liking.
6. Strain (Optional):
   a. If you prefer a smoother tea, you can strain out the ginger slices and mint leaves at this point.
7. Refrigerate:
   a. Place the iced ginger mint green tea in the refrigerator for at least 1-2 hours to allow the flavors to meld.
8. Serve Over Ice:
   a. Fill glasses with ice cubes and pour the chilled tea over the ice.
9. Garnish (Optional):
   a. Garnish with lemon slices for a citrusy touch.
10. Stir and Enjoy:
    a. Give the Iced Ginger Mint Green Tea a gentle stir and enjoy this refreshing and

flavorful iced tea.

Note:

• Experiment with the ginger and mint quantities to adjust the intensity of flavors.

• This tea can be prepared in larger batches for gatherings or parties.

Nutrition Information (Approximate Values):

• Calories: 10

• Carbohydrates: 2g

• Sugars: 1g

• Sodium: 5mg

CITRUS INFUSED SPA WATER

Spa Water Description:

This Citrus Infused Spa Water is a refreshing and hydrating drink that adds a burst of citrusy flavors to your water. Packed with the goodness of fruits and herbs, this spa water is delicious and a healthy way to stay hydrated throughout the day.

Ingredients:

• One orange, thinly sliced

• One lemon, thinly sliced

• One lime, thinly sliced

• One grapefruit, thinly sliced

• Handful of fresh mint leaves

• Ice cubes

• Water

Instructions:

1. Prepare Citrus Slices:
   a. Wash and thinly slice the orange, lemon, lime, and grapefruit. Ensure the slices are thin for better infusion.
2. Add Citrus Slices to Pitcher:

       a. Place the citrus slices in a large pitcher.
3. Add Fresh Mint:
       a. Add a handful of fresh mint leaves to the pitcher. Crush the mint gently with a spoon to release its flavor.
4. Fill the Pitcher with Water:
       a. Fill the pitcher with cold water. For a more enhanced flavor, you can use sparkling water.
5. Stir Gently:
       a. Give the ingredients in the pitcher a gentle stir to distribute the flavors.
6. Refrigerate:
       a. Refrigerate the Citrus Infused Spa Water for at least 1-2 hours to allow the flavors to infuse into the water.
7. Serve Over Ice:
       a. Fill glasses with ice cubes and pour the infused spa water over the ice.
8. Garnish (Optional):
       a. Garnish individual glasses with additional citrus slices or mint leaves for a decorative touch.
9. Enjoy:
       a. Enjoy this Citrus Infused Spa Water as a refreshing and hydrating beverage.

Note:

• For varied flavors, experiment with different citrus fruits or herbs like basil or rosemary.

• The infused water can be kept in the refrigerator for up to 24 hours.

Nutrition Information (Approximate Values):

- Calories: 10
- Carbohydrates: 3g
- Sugars: 2g
- Sodium: 2mg

FRESH ORANGE AND CARROT JUICE

Juice Description:

This Fresh Orange and Carrot Juice is a vibrant and nutrient-packed drink that combines the sweet and citrusy flavor of oranges with the earthy sweetness of carrots. Packed with vitamins and antioxidants, this juice tastes refreshing and provides a healthy boost to your immune system.

Ingredients:

• Four large oranges, peeled and segmented

• Four medium-sized carrots, peeled and chopped

• Ice cubes (optional)

Instructions:

1. Prepare Ingredients:
   a. Peel the oranges and separate them into segments. Peel and chop the carrots into smaller pieces for easier juicing.
2. Juice Oranges and Carrots:
   a. Juice the peeled and segmented oranges and chopped carrots using a juicer. If you don't have a juicer, you can use a blender and strain the mixture to

extract the juice.

3. Strain (Optional):

    a. If using a blender, strain the juice using a fine mesh sieve or cheesecloth to remove the pulp. This step is optional, depending on your preference for pulp in the juice.

4. Chill (Optional):

    a. Refrigerate the Fresh Orange and Carrot Juice for 30 minutes or serve it immediately over ice.

5. Serve:

    a. Pour the juice into glasses.

6. Garnish (Optional):

    a. Garnish with a slice of orange on the rim of the glass or a sprig of mint for a decorative touch.

7. Enjoy:

    a. Enjoy this revitalizing Fresh Orange and Carrot Juice as a nutritious and delicious beverage.

Note:

• Adjust the sweetness by adding a touch of honey or agave syrup if desired.

• Experiment with adding a small piece of ginger for a zesty kick.

Nutrition Information (Approximate Values):

• Calories: 120

• Carbohydrates: 28g

• Sugars: 20g

- Protein: 2g
- Fiber: 5g
- Fat: 0.5g
- Sodium: 80mg

WATERMELON GAZPACHO WITH MINT

Gazpacho Description:

This Watermelon Gazpacho with Mint is a refreshing and hydrating twist on the classic Spanish soup. The juicy sweetness of watermelon is combined with the vibrant flavors of tomatoes, cucumber, and mint, creating a delightful chilled soup perfect for hot days.

Ingredients:

- 4 cups seedless watermelon, diced
- Two large tomatoes, diced
- One cucumber, peeled and diced
- One red bell pepper, diced
- 1/4 red onion, finely chopped
- Two tablespoons fresh mint, chopped
- Two tablespoons extra-virgin olive oil
- Three tablespoons of red wine vinegar
- Salt and black pepper to taste
- 1 cup cold water (adjust for desired consistency)

• Ice cubes (optional)

Instructions:

1. Prepare Ingredients:
   a. Dice the watermelon, tomatoes, cucumber, and red bell pepper into uniform pieces. Finely chop the red onion and fresh mint.
2. Blend Ingredients:
   a. Combine the diced watermelon, tomatoes, cucumber, red bell pepper, red onion, and mint in a blender.
3. Add Olive Oil and Vinegar:
   a. Pour in the extra-virgin olive oil and red wine vinegar.
4. Season and Blend:
   a. Season with salt and black pepper to taste. Blend the ingredients until smooth.
5. Adjust Consistency:
   a. If the gazpacho is too thick, add cold water in small amounts until you achieve the desired consistency. Blend again to incorporate.
6. Chill:
   a. Refrigerate the Watermelon Gazpacho for at least 1-2 hours to allow the flavors to meld and the soup to chill.
7. Serve Cold:
   a. Ladle the chilled gazpacho into bowls. If desired, add ice cubes to each serving for an extra chill.
8. Garnish (Optional):

      a. Garnish with additional chopped mint before serving.

9. Enjoy:

      a. Enjoy this refreshing Watermelon Gazpacho with Mint as an excellent and revitalizing appetizer or light meal.

Note:

• Customize the gazpacho by adjusting the quantity of mint or adding a touch of lime juice for extra zest.

• This soup can be made ahead of time and stored in the refrigerator for a day.

Nutrition Information (Approximate Values):

• Calories: 150

• Carbohydrates: 25g

• Sugars: 18g

• Protein: 2g

• Fat: 7g

• Fiber: 4g

• Sodium: 150mg

SPARKLING BERRY LEMONADE

Lemonade Description:

This Sparkling Berry Lemonade is a fizzy and refreshing twist on the classic lemonade, featuring a burst of mixed berries. It's a perfect thirst-quencher for hot days or a delightful beverage for any occasion.

Ingredients:

• 1 cup mixed berries (strawberries, blueberries, raspberries)

• 1 cup freshly squeezed lemon juice (about 4-6 lemons)

• 1/2 cup granulated sugar (adjust to taste)

• 4 cups cold sparkling water

• Ice cubes

• Lemon slices and mixed berries for garnish

• Fresh mint leaves for garnish (optional)

Instructions:

1. Prepare Mixed Berries:
    a. Wash and prepare the mixed berries. If using strawberries, hull and slice them.
2. Make Berry Puree:
    a. In a blender, puree the mixed berries

until smooth. Strain the puree to remove seeds if desired.

3. Mix Lemonade Base:

   a. In a pitcher, combine the freshly squeezed lemon juice and granulated sugar. Stir until the sugar is dissolved.

4. Add Berry Puree:

   a. Add the berry puree to the lemonade base. Mix well to combine.

5. Add Sparkling Water:

   a. Pour in the cold sparkling water. Stir gently to incorporate the sparkling water into the lemonade mixture.

6. Taste and Adjust:

   a. Taste the Sparkling Berry Lemonade and adjust the sweetness by adding more sugar if needed.

7. Chill:

   a. Refrigerate the lemonade for at least 1-2 hours to allow the flavors to meld and the mixture to chill.

8. Serve Over Ice:

   a. Fill glasses with ice cubes and pour the Sparkling Berry Lemonade over the ice.

9. Garnish:

   a. Garnish each glass with lemon slices, mixed berries, and fresh mint leaves if desired.

10. Enjoy:

   a. Enjoy this delightful Sparkling Berry Lemonade as a bubbly and fruity treat.

Note:

- Experiment with different berry combinations for varied flavors.

- Add a splash of your favorite clear spirit, like vodka or gin, for an adult version.

Nutrition Information (Approximate Values):

- Calories: 120
- Carbohydrates: 30g
- Sugars: 22g
- Protein: 1g
- Sodium: 20mg

WATERMELON AND MINT COOLER

Cooler Description:

This Watermelon and Mint Cooler is a refreshing and hydrating beverage that combines the natural sweetness of watermelon with the invigorating flavor of fresh mint. This cooler is a delightful way to stay calm and quench your thirst, perfect for hot summer days.

Ingredients:

• 4 cups seedless watermelon, diced

• 1/4 cup fresh mint leaves

• Two tablespoons of lime juice

• Two tablespoons honey or agave syrup (adjust to taste)

• 2 cups cold water

• Ice cubes

• Mint sprigs and watermelon wedges for garnish

Instructions:

1. Prepare Watermelon:
    a. Dice the seedless watermelon into small cubes, removing any seeds.
2. Blend Watermelon and Mint:
    a. In a blender, combine the diced

watermelon and fresh mint leaves. Blend until smooth.

3. Strain (Optional):
   a. If you prefer a smoother texture, strain the blended mixture using a fine mesh sieve or cheesecloth to remove pulp.
4. Add Lime Juice and Sweetener:
   a. Add lime juice and honey (or agave syrup) to the watermelon-mint mixture. Adjust the sweetness to your liking.
5. Mix with Cold Water:
   a. In a pitcher, combine the watermelon-mint blend with cold water. Stir well to mix.
6. Chill:
   a. Refrigerate the Watermelon and Mint Cooler for at least 1-2 hours to enhance the flavors and chill the drink.
7. Serve Over Ice:
   a. Fill glasses with ice cubes and pour the cooled cooler over the ice.
8. Garnish:
   a. Garnish each glass with a sprig of mint and a small watermelon wedge for a decorative touch.
9. Stir and Enjoy:
   a. Give the cooler a gentle stir and enjoy this refreshing Watermelon and Mint Cooler.
10. Note:
    a. For an extra chill, you can freeze some watermelon cubes and use them as ice

cubes in the cooler.

b. Customize by adding a splash of sparkling water for some effervescence.

Nutrition Information (Approximate Values):

- Calories: 80

- Carbohydrates: 20g

- Sugars: 16g

- Protein: 1g

- Sodium: 5mg

COCONUT WATER SMOOTHIE WITH PINEAPPLE AND MANGO

Smoothie Description:

This Coconut Water Smoothie with Pineapple and Mango is a tropical and hydrating blend that combines the electrolyte-rich goodness of coconut water with the vibrant flavors of pineapple and mango. Packed with vitamins and minerals, this smoothie is a refreshing and nutritious choice for a quick pick-me-up.

Ingredients:

- 1 cup coconut water
- 1 cup frozen pineapple chunks
- 1 cup frozen mango chunks
- One banana, peeled and sliced
- 1/2 cup Greek yogurt (optional for creaminess)
- One tablespoon of chia seeds (optional for added nutrition)
- Ice cubes (optional)

Instructions:

1. Add Coconut Water:
   a. Pour coconut water into a blender as the base for the smoothie.
2. Add Frozen Fruits:
   a. Add frozen pineapple chunks and frozen mango chunks to the blender.
3. Include Banana:
   a. Add the sliced banana to the other ingredients in the blender.
4. Optional Greek Yogurt:
   a. If you desire a creamier texture, add Greek yogurt to the blender.
5. Optional Chia Seeds:
   a. For an extra nutritional boost, include chia seeds in the blender.
6. Blend Until Smooth:
   a. Blend all the ingredients until smooth and creamy. If the smoothie is too thick, add more coconut or a bit of regular water.
7. Check Consistency:
   a. Adjust the consistency by adding ice cubes if a colder and icier texture is preferred.
8. Pour and Serve:
   a. Pour the Coconut Water Smoothie into glasses.
9. Garnish (Optional):
   a. Garnish with a slice of pineapple or a wedge of mango on the rim of the glass.
10. Enjoy:
    a. Enjoy this tropical and hydrating

Coconut Water Smoothie with Pineapple and Mango as a delicious and nutritious beverage.

Note:

• Experiment with different frozen fruits for varied flavors.

• Customize the sweetness by adjusting the amount of banana or adding a touch of honey if desired.

Nutrition Information (Approximate Values):

• Calories: 200

• Carbohydrates: 45g

• Sugars: 30g

• Protein: 4g

• Fat: 2g

• Fiber: 7g

• Sodium: 50mg

HERBAL ICED TEA WITH LEMON AND HONEY

Iced Tea Description:

This Herbal Iced Tea with Lemon and Honey is a refreshing and soothing beverage that combines the flavors of herbal tea, citrusy lemons, and the natural sweetness of honey. It's a perfect way to cool down on a hot day or enjoy a calming drink.

Ingredients:

• Four herbal tea bags (chamomile, peppermint, or your choice)

• 4 cups boiling water

• One lemon, sliced

• 2-3 tablespoons honey (adjust to taste)

• Ice cubes

• Fresh mint leaves for garnish (optional)

Instructions:

    1. Brew Herbal Tea:

        a. Place the herbal tea bags in a heatproof pitcher. Pour boiling water over the tea

bags and let them steep for 5-7 minutes.
2. Sweeten with Honey:
    a. Add honey to the hot tea and stir until it dissolves. Adjust the sweetness according to your preference.
3. Cool Tea:
    a. Allow the tea to cool to room temperature. You can speed up the process by placing it in the refrigerator.
4. Add Lemon Slices:
    a. Once the tea has cooled, add slices of lemon to the pitcher. Stir gently.
5. Refrigerate:
    a. Refrigerate the Herbal Iced Tea for at least 1-2 hours to enhance the flavors and chill the drink.
6. Serve Over Ice:
    a. Fill glasses with ice cubes and pour the chilled tea over the ice.
7. Garnish (Optional):
    a. Garnish each glass with a sprig of fresh mint leaves for freshness.
8. Stir and Enjoy:
    a. Give the tea a gentle stir and enjoy this Herbal Iced Tea with Lemon and Honey as a refreshing and calming beverage.

Note:

• Experiment with different herbal tea blends for unique flavors.

• Adjust the amount of honey and lemon to suit your taste preferences.

Nutrition Information (Approximate Values):

- Calories: 20
- Carbohydrates: 6g
- Sugars: 5g
- Protein: 0g
- Fat: 0g
- Sodium: 5mg

INFUSED WATER WITH CUCUMBER AND MINT

Infused Water Description:

This Infused Water with Cucumber and Mint is a simple yet refreshing way to add natural flavor to your water. The coolness of cucumber, combined with the invigorating taste of mint, creates a delightful beverage that is both hydrating and enjoyable.

Ingredients:

- 1/2 cucumber, thinly sliced
- Handful of fresh mint leaves
- One lemon, thinly sliced (optional)
- Ice cubes
- 4 cups cold water

Instructions:

1. Prepare Ingredients:
    a. Wash the cucumber thoroughly and cut it into thin slices. Rinse the mint leaves.
2. Assemble in a Pitcher:
    a. In a large pitcher, combine the

cucumber slices and fresh mint leaves. If desired, add thin slices of lemon for an extra citrusy flavor.

3. Muddle (Optional):
   a. Gently muddle the cucumber and mint with a wooden spoon to release their flavors. This step is optional but enhances the infusion.

4. Add Cold Water:
   a. Pour cold water into the pitcher over the cucumber and mint. Stir gently to combine.

5. Refrigerate:
   a. Refrigerate the Infused Water for at least 1-2 hours to allow the flavors to infuse into the water.

6. Serve Over Ice:
   a. Fill glasses with ice cubes and pour the infused water over the ice.

7. Garnish (Optional):
   a. Garnish individual glasses with additional cucumber slices, mint leaves, or lemon slices for a decorative touch.

8. Stir and Enjoy:
   a. Give the infused water a gentle stir before sipping, and enjoy the crisp and refreshing taste of Cucumber and Mint Infused Water.

Note:

• Experiment with different variations, such as adding a handful of berries or a splash of sparkling water.

• You can add a touch of honey or agave syrup for a

sweeter option.

Nutrition Information (Approximate Values):

- Calories: 0
- Carbohydrates: 0g
- Sugars: 0g
- Protein: 0g
- Fat: 0g
- Sodium: 0mg

CONCLUSION

In conclusion, the intricate interplay between diet and dementia underscores the significance of adopting a proactive and informed approach to support cognitive health. As we grapple with the increasing prevalence of dementia in an aging global population, understanding the potential impact of dietary habits on brain function has become paramount. The exploration of nutritional patterns, nutrients, and lifestyle choices has provided valuable insights into strategies that may contribute to the preservation of cognitive abilities and the potential delay of cognitive decline.

However, it is crucial to approach the role of diet in dementia with a nuanced perspective. While dietary interventions offer a promising avenue for promoting brain health, they should be seen as part of a comprehensive approach that includes other lifestyle factors such as regular physical activity, mental stimulation, and social engagement. Moreover, individualized guidance from healthcare professionals and registered dietitians is essential to tailor dietary recommendations to specific health needs and conditions.

As we continue to unravel the complexities of dementia and its relationship with diet, it is imperative to acknowledge that no single solution exists. Dementia is a multifaceted condition influenced by various factors, including genetics and overall health. While embracing a brain-healthy diet is a proactive step, it is equally important to foster a broader societal awareness, dispel stigmas associated with dementia, and invest in research that expands our understanding of preventive strategies.